Diagnostic Imaging of Ophthalmology

Zhenchang Wang • Junfang Xian
Fengyuan Man • Zhengyu Zhang
Editors

Diagnostic Imaging of Ophthalmology

A Practical Atlas

人民軍醫出版社
PEOPLE'S MILITARY MEDICAL PRESS

Springer

Editors
Zhenchang Wang
Beijing Friendship Hospital Capital Medical University
Beijing
China

Junfang Xian
Beijing Tongren Hospital Capital Medical University
Beijing
China

Fengyuan Man
PLA Rocket Force General Hospital
Beijing
China

Zhengyu Zhang
Department of Radiology
Beijing Unicare ENT Hospital
Beijing
China

ISBN 978-94-024-1058-7 ISBN 978-94-024-1060-0 (eBook)
https://doi.org/10.1007/978-94-024-1060-0
The print edition is not for sale in China Mainland. Customers from China Mainland please order the print book from: People's Military Medical Press.

Library of Congress Control Number: 2017952040

Printed on acid-free paper

This Springer imprint is published by Springer Nature
The registered company is Springer Science+Business Media B.V.
The registered company address is: Van Godewijckstraat 30, 3311 GX Dordrecht, The Netherlands

Preface

With the advances in medicine, the understanding of eye disorders has been improving and deepening. In the meanwhile, imaging exam plays an increasingly important role in the diagnosis of ophthalmic diseases. For young radiologists, the training and improvement of imaging diagnosis thinking as well as the accumulation of practical experience is a must process. In addition, with the imaging technique development and the increasing application, new imaging techniques play a more and more important, sometimes even indispensable, role in the clinical diagnosis and treatment of ophthalmic diseases, and accordingly ophthalmologists show unprecedented attention and interest in these technologies, having a strong demand for knowledge updates.

Ophthalmology service in Beijing Tongren Hospital, Capital Medical University, is the ace specialty in China, and its ophthalmic imaging exams and diagnostic capabilities rank in the leading level throughout the country. With an aim to introduce our experience to more peers, we've summarized the images of common ophthalmic diseases collected in Beijing Tongren Hospital during recent years, and compiled this book of our experience in selecting imaging methods, imaging diagnosis, and differential diagnosis in ophthalmic diseases.

In view of the target readers of this book, we try to make this book: (1) Systematic—This book, based on common diseases and written by anatomical sites, briefly describes the pathology, clinical characteristics, selection of imaging method, imaging diagnosis, and differential diagnosis. (2) Practical—This book has the *Comment* part at the end of each section, which focuses on providing summaries and tips on choosing imaging techniques, imaging exam and diagnosis key points, and things that should be paid special attention to. (3) Readable—Images in this book are well displayed and equipped with the detailed illustrations. For main structures and lesion details shown in the pictures, eye-catching marks are added. The small size of this book makes it easy for readers to carry and look up in the clinical work.

Due to the limited preparation time, we believe that there should be some inevitable errors and omissions in this book. We earnestly hope that our readers would not hesitate to point them out to us and make this book better and better.

Beijing, China Zhenchang Wang
Beijing, China Junfang Xian
Beijing, China Fengyuan Man
Beijing, China Zhengyu Zhang

Contents

Chapter 1
Imaging Methods Commonly Used for Orbit Examination and the Normal Imaging Presentations

Weidi Ming, Fengyuan Man, and Zhengyu Zhang

1.1 X-ray

X-ray examination for orbit is easy to perform and with low price; however, this method also has many limitations and thus the diagnostic value is limited. Currently, X-ray examination for orbit is mainly used for ruling out or locating orbital foreign body and dacryocystography, while the other orbital disorders are generally diagnosed with ultrasound, CT, and MRI. In addition, CT scanning has also been widely used for ruling out or locating orbital foreign body instead of X-ray currently, as CT scanning could better display the size, location, and relationships of the foreign body with adjacent tissues (Rose 1993).

1.1.1 Normal Presentations on Orbital X-ray Images

1. Posteroanterior images of orbit and the presentations: On posteroanterior X-ray images, the margin of orbit in adults is shown as a rectangle structure tended to be oval, while the orbital margin in infants tended to be round, but the structures are not as clear as in adults, and the percentage in facial bone is relatively large. The superior wall of orbit is the base of anterior cranial fossa. The posteroanterior X-ray image shows that there is a crescent-shaped high-density shadow at the outer margin of the orbit; the white line at the upper margin represents the projection of the lacrimal fossa roof, while the white line at the lower margin is the projection of the upper orbital margin. The X-ray image of medial orbit wall mainly shows 2–3 high-density lines. The inferior orbit wall is the upper wall of

W. Ming • F. Man (✉)
Department of Medical Imaging, The PLA Rocket Force General Hospital, Beijing, China
e-mail: manfengyuan@yeah.net

Z. Zhang
Department of Radiology, Beijing Unicare ENT Hospital, Beijing, China

Z. Wang et al. (eds.), *Diagnostic Imaging of Ophthalmology*,
https://doi.org/10.1007/978-94-024-1060-0_1

maxillary sinus, which is very thin and is displayed as fine linear shadow that slightly concave upward on the posteroanterior X-ray image. The lateral orbit wall is the boundary between orbit and temporal fossa. The anterior part of the lateral orbit wall is mainly composed of the angular process of frontal bone and frontal process of zygomatic bone, while the posterior part is composed of the greater wing of sphenoid bone. On posteroanterior X-ray images, the lateral orbit wall is leaning backward and thus could not be clearly displayed. Most part of the posterior orbit wall is composed of sphenoid bone; the superior orbital fissure is the boundary between the upper orbit wall and lateral orbit wall, and inferior orbital fissure is the boundary between inferior orbit wall and lateral orbit wall. On posteroanterior X-ray images, the superior orbital fissure is shown as the transparent clearance between superior orbit wall and lateral orbit wall, while the inferior orbital fissure could not be displayed (Fig. 1.1a).

2. Lateral images of orbit and the presentations: On lateral X-ray images, the bilateral orbits are overlapped. Most part of the superior orbit wall is the horizontal part of frontal bone, and the tissues above orbits are the base of anterior cranial fossa, which are shown as high-density wavy linear shadows, while the lower margin is very smooth. The bilateral lesser wings of sphenoid bones overlapped, and the medial end is the anterior clinoid process. The anterior margin of lateral orbit wall is shown as thick linear shadow that slightly concave forward, while the posterior orbit wall is shown as two nearly parallel linear shadows at the space orbit apex that slightly protrude forward. The bone at the orbit floor is very thin, and maxillary sinus could be found below the orbit floor (Fig. 1.1b).

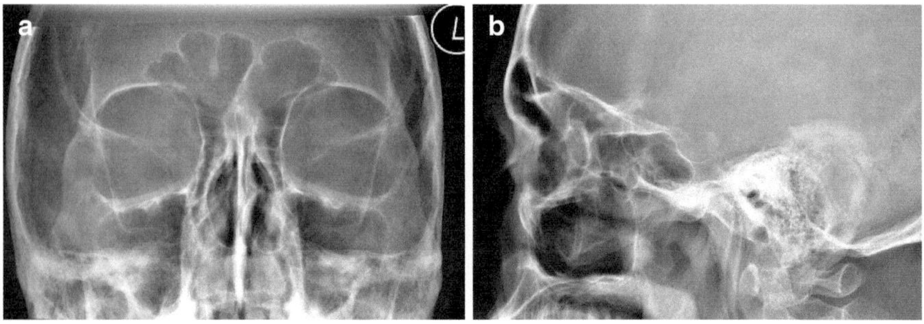

Fig. 1.1 Normal images of orbit. (**a**) Posteroanterior, (**b**) lateral

1.1.2 Normal X-ray Presentations on Dacryocystography

Dacryocystography is used to explore the shape, size, and obstruction (including the severity and location of obstruction) of dacryocyst. Iodine allergy test is required for the patients receiving dacryocystography. The normal nasolacrimal duct is unobstructed; thus, contrast agent could flow to inferior meatus rapidly, and only small amount of contrast agent could be found in the regions of dacryocyst and nasolacrimal duct; in addition, contrast agent could also be found in nasal cavity (Fig. 1.2).

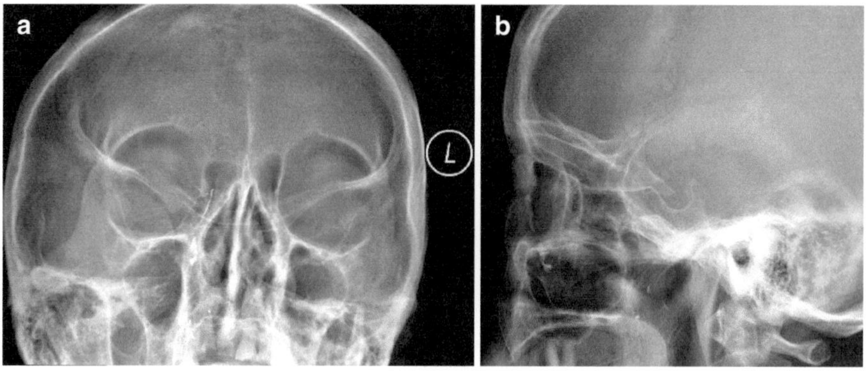

Fig. 1.2 Dacryocystography of the right side. (**a**) Posteroanterior, (**b**) lateral

1.2 Computed Tomography (CT)

CT scanning is the most commonly used technology for the examinations of orbit, which could clearly display the anatomic structures, especially the bony structures in ocular region. For the patients with traumatic injuries, three-dimensional CT scanning could directly display the shape of the orbital injuries and thus helps deciding operation plan.

Currently, multi-row spiral CT scanning is routinely used for the CT scanning of orbit, after which the raw images are used for multi-planar reconstruction. Cross-sectional and coronary images are the most commonly reconstructed images. For the patients with posterior orbit wall lesions or postocular lesions, oblique sagittal reconstruction is an effective supplement (Goh et al. 2008). The anatomic features of orbit at the major levels on CT images are described as follows (Fig. 1.3):

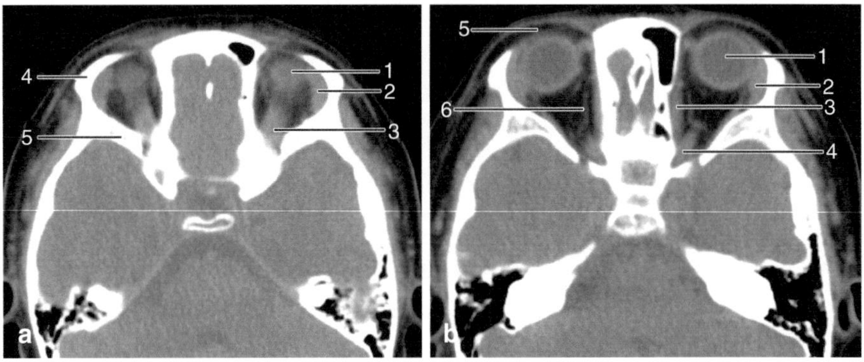

Fig. 1.3 The normal orbit by CT scan (Axial CT (**a–d**), Coronal CT (**e–i**), Coronal CT (bone window) (**j–l**), Sagittal CT (**m, n**)). (**a**) *1* superior of the eyeball, *2* lacrimal gland, *3* superior rectus, *4* superior margin of the orbit, *5* posterolateral wall of the orbit; (**b**) *1* eyeball, *2* lacrimal gland, *3* medial rectus, *4* optic nerve, 5 eyelid, *6* ophthalmic artery; (**c**) *1* atria, *2* lens, *3* vitreum, *4* optic nerve, *5* lateral rectus, *6* superior orbital fissure, *7* lacrimal gland, *8* media rectus; (**d**) *1* atria, *2* vitreum, *3* inferior rectus, *4* inferior orbital fissure, *5* pterygopalatine fossa, *6* lens, *7* media rectus, *8* posterolateral wall of the orbit, *9* greater wing of sphenoid bone; (**e**) *1* vitreum, *2* lens, *3* lacrimal sac area, *4* orbital process of frontal bone, *5* eye thimble; (**f**) *1* lacrimal gland, *2* vitreum, *3* the insertion of media rectus, *4* inferior obliquus, *5* nasolacrimal duct, *6* the insertion of superior rectus, *7* the insertion of lateral rectus, *8* the insertion of inferior rectus; (**g**) *1* superior muscle group of orbit, *2* lacrimal gland, *3* vitreum, *4* inferior rectus, *5* superior obliquus, *6* media rectus; (**h**) *1* superior muscle group of orbit, *2* superior ophthalmic vein, *3* superior obliquus, *4* media rectus, *5* inferior rectus, *6* ophthalmic artery, *7* optic nerve, *8* lateral rectus, *9* infraorbital canal; (**i**) *1* anterior clinoid process, *2* orbital apex, *3* inferior orbital fissure, *4* pterygopalatine fossa, *5* lesser wing of sphenoid bone, *6* superior orbital fissure, *7* greater wing of sphenoid bone, *8* sphenoid sinus, *9* pterygomaxillary fissure; (**j**) *1* frontal sinus, *2* paries superior orbitae, *3* the upper inner corner of paries superior orbitae, *4* ethmoidal sinus, *5* the lower inner corner of paries inferior orbitae, *6* nasolacrimal duct, *7* maxillary sinus; (**k**) *1* optic canal, *2* anterior clinoid process, *3* greater wing of sphenoid bone, *4* foramen rotundum, *5* sphenoid sinus, *6* the superior wall of optic canal, *7* superior orbital fissure, *8* orbital apex, *9* medial and lower wall of optic canal; (**l**) *1* optic canal, *2* anterior clinoid process, *3* orbital apex, *4* foramen rotundum, *5* sphenoid sinus, *6* planum sphenoidale, *7* middle cranial fossa, *8* greater wing of sphenoid bone, *9* vidian canal, *10* processes sphenoid bone pterygoid; (**m**) *1* lacrimal gland, *2* vitreum, *3* lateral rectus, *4* maxillary sinus; (**n**) *1* superior muscle group of the orbit, *2* optic nerve, *3* anterior chamber, *4* lens, *5* vitreum, *6* inferior rectus

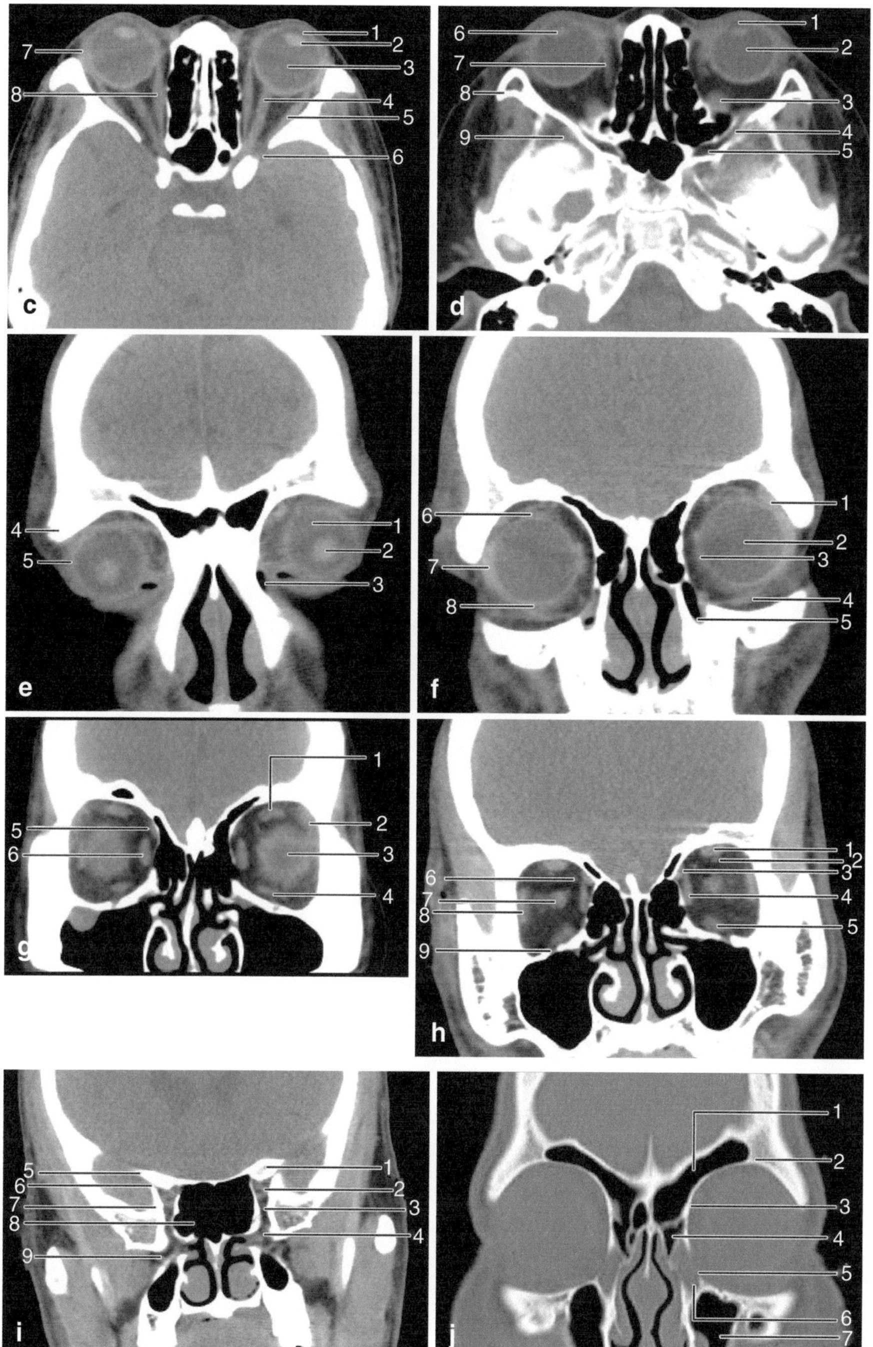

Fig. 1.3 (continued)

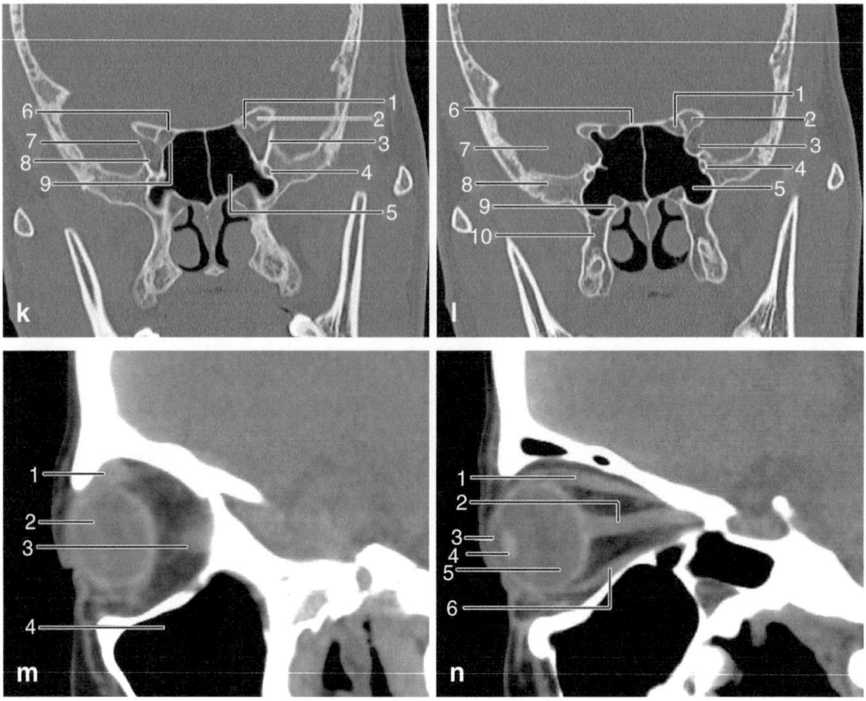

Fig. 1.3 (continued)

1.3 Magnetic Resonance Imaging (MRI)

Magnetic resonance imaging (MRI) is now commonly used for the imaging examinations of orbit, which has more advantages to display soft tissue lesions than CT. In addition to conventional examination sequences, using other new technologies (such as fat suppression technique) appropriately could help avoiding chemical shift artifacts and thus clearly displaying the lesions.

As the anatomic images of MRI are similar to CT images, only the MRI images of normal orbit at several levels are described here (Fig. 1.4).

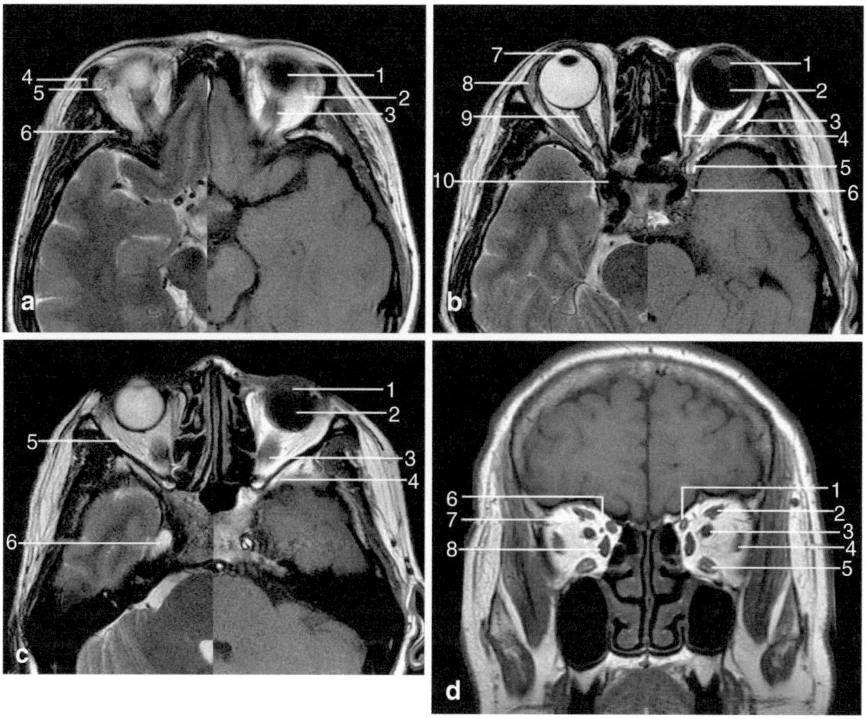

Fig. 1.4 The normal orbit by MRI, (**a**–**c**) Axial (L T2WI, R:T1WI) (**d**) Coronal (T1WI). (**a**) *1* vitreum, *2* fat in orbital cavity, *3* superior muscle group of the orbit, *4* orbital process of frontal bone, *5* lacrimal gland, *6* greater wing of sphenoid bone; (**b**) *1* lens, *2* vitreum, *3* lateral rectus, *4* medial rectus, *5* superior orbital fissure, *6* cavernous sinus, *7* atria, *8* lacrimal gland, *9* optic nerve, *10* internal carotid artery; (**c**) *1* lens, *2* vitreum, *3* inferior rectus, *4* greater wing of sphenoid bone, *5* fat in orbital cavity, *6* Meckel's cave; (**d**) *1* superior obliquus, *2* superior rectus, *3* optic nerve, *4* lateral rectus, *5* inferior rectus, *6* ophthalmic artery, *7* superior ophthalmic vein, *8* medial rectus

1.4 Ultrasound Examinations and Radionuclide Imaging

1.4.1 Ultrasound

Ultrasound examinations are very sensitive for identifying retinopathy and intraocular lesions. Type A ultrasound examination is mainly used for the measurement of biological values of the eyeball in clinical practices, which is a routine examination before intraocular lens implantation. While type B ultrasound examination could dynamically display the location, size, and shape of the lesion, as well as the relationships with adjacent tissues, and has been accepted as the routine imaging method for examination and screening of ocular lesions. Color Doppler imaging overlays the color blood flow characteristics on type B gray-scale images, and could be used to examine the blood flow in ophthalmic artery, central retinal artery, and posterior ciliary artery, as well as blood supply for ocular lesions. Ultrasound examinations are also helpful for localizing and qualitative diagnosing tumors; however, the specificity of ultrasound examination is very low, and the post-ocular lesions could not be diagnosed. In addition, the range of extraocular and extraorbital invasion could not be correctly displayed, and thus ultrasound examination could only be used as a screening method. For orbital lesions, there are only few indications for ultrasound examinations. The display of small lesions and overall anatomic structures of ultrasound examination is not as good as CT or MRI (Udani and Bury 2013).

1.4.2 Radionuclide Imaging

For the cases with orbital tumors, the tumor operations and radiotherapy could induce the scar formation and anatomic structure distortion; therefore, it is very difficult to identify residual tumors or tumor recurrence by conventional imaging methods, especially within 1 year after the operation. In contrast, PET has unique value in diagnosing the posttreatment recurrence and evaluating treatment efficacies on orbital tumors, which could identify the tumor recurrence and residual tumors (Krassas and Kahaly 1999). However, the resolution of PET on anatomic structures is relatively low, which restricted the application of this method in identifying and localizing tumors; in addition, the insufficient spatial resolution also limited the value of PET in diagnosing small tumors; furthermore, PET scanning is relatively expensive, and only few major hospitals have the PET scanning system. Therefore, efforts are needed for the wide application of PET scanning.

References

Goh PS, Gi MT, Charlton A, et al. Review of orbital imaging. Eur J Radiol. 2008;66(3):387–95.

Krassas GE, Kahaly GJ. The role of octreoscan in thyroid eye disease. Eur J Endocrinol. 1999;140(5):373–5.

Rose GE. Orbital imaging. Curr Opin Ophthalmol. 1993;4(5):70–5.

Udani SD, Bury RW. Transverse ultrasound image through the orbit. BMJ. 2013;347(Supplement):f6780.

Chapter 2
Ocular Developmental Lesions

Pengfei Zhao, Zhenchang Wang, and Zhengyu Zhang

2.1 Congenital Anophthalmia

Congenital anophthalmia is known as a rare congenital disease clinically. It is divided into two types according to the pathogenesis and organizational form: (1) primary anophthalmia: it is thought to be caused by the chromosome aberration in the early embryo (within 3 weeks), which results in underdevelopment of the optic vesicle or optic pit in the orbit. (2) Secondary anophthalmia: the optic vesicle is formed in the early embryo but degenerates due to some exogenous or endogenous causes, and thus the intact eyeball is failed to be formed.

2.1.1 Pathological Features

1. Congenital anophthalmia: No structure originated from the optic vesicle exists in the orbit, usually accompanied by deformity of the optic canal and normal development of the eyelid, conjunctiva, eye muscle, and orbit.
2. Secondary anophthalmia: Dysplastic or embryonic tissues originated from the optic vesicle, such as retina, pigment, and retinal pigment epithelium, can be found in the orbit.

P. Zhao • Z. Wang (✉)
Department of Radiology, Beijing Friendship Hospital, Capital Medical University, Beijing, China
e-mail: cjr.wzhch@vip.163.com

Z. Zhang
Department of Radiology, Beijing Unicare ENT Hospital, Beijing, China

Z. Wang et al. (eds.), *Diagnostic Imaging of Ophthalmology*,
https://doi.org/10.1007/978-94-024-1060-0_2

3. Anophthalmia and severe microphthalmia: It is difficult to distinguish the two diseases clinically. Primary anophthalmus can be identified only after serial section examination of all the orbital tissues with no ectodermal tissues found. However, it is impossible to identify the diagnosis according to orbital pathology due to various causes; therefore, both conditions are referred to as "primary anophthalmus" (Davies 2007).

2.1.2 *Imaging Examination*

1. CT: It is considered as the first choice of the examination for this disease.
2. MRI: When CT is unable to distinguish whether the soft tissue is an accessory structure of the residual eyeball structure or not, or it is necessary to eliminate other concomitant lesions, MRI of orbit should be performed.

2.1.3 *Imaging Performance*

1. X-ray performance: Patients with no eyeball or severe small eyeball can be seen with soft tissue in the small and round orbital fossa. The ipsilateral orbital bone and optic foramen are generally small, even absent.
2. CT performance: The orbit is usually small with no eyeball or irregular soft-tissue mass. The accessory structures such as the extraocular muscles and optic nerve are usually slender (Figs. 2.1 and 2.2).
3. MRI performance: Irregular soft tissue can be seen in the portion of absent eyeball, which is iso-intense on T1WI and heterogeneous iso- or hypo-intense on T2WI, and with no obvious enhancement.

2.1.4 *Evaluation*

The clinical symptoms of patients with congenital anophthalmia are obvious and diagnosis can be easily made after clinical examination. In order to have a more detailed understanding of the disease, ultrasound or CT examinations can be further performed. If the density of soft tissue in the orbit is heterogeneous and its boundary with surrounding structures is not clear, MRI examination should be further performed to exclude neoplastic lesions.

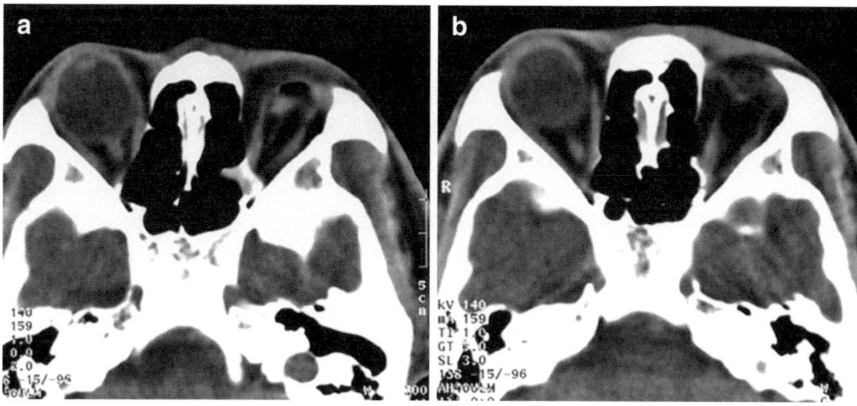

Fig. 2.1 Left congenital anophthalmia. (**a**) Axial CT scan shows that the left orbital cavity becomes smaller with no normal eyeball, where irregular nodular soft tissue can be seen. In addition, medial rectus, lateral rectus, and optic nerve are slender. The right eyeball becomes bigger with fronted lens and shallow anterior chamber. (**b**) Axial CT scan is the upper section of the (**a**), which shows smaller left orbital cavity and irregular soft tissue in the portion of absent eyeball

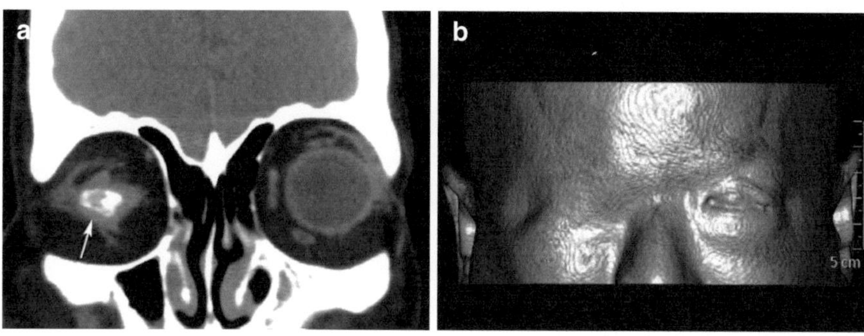

Fig. 2.2 Right congenital anophthalmia. (**a**) Coronal CT scan shows that the right orbital cavity becomes smaller with irregular hyper-dense soft tissue in the portion of absent eyeball. In addition, the extraocular muscles become slender. (**b**) 3D CT scan shows no palpebral fissure deformity on the right side and slightly sunken eye fossa

2.2 Congenital Microphthalmia

There are three types of microphthalmia: deficient microphthalmia, concurrent microphthalmia, and simple microphthalmia. Simple microphthalmia means that the volume of the eyeball is smaller but with no other significant ocular deformities. Deficient microphthalmia refers to the congenital defect of ocular tissue in embryonic stage. Concurrent microphthalmia means small eyeball with other ocular malformations, in which a persistent hyperplasia of the primary vitreous (PHPV) is most common.

2.2.1 *Pathological Features*

1. Simple microphthalmia manifests as slightly smaller eyeball, resulting from growth stagnation in late embryo.
2. The internal structure of the eyeball is generally normal; the orbital volume decreases slightly and the lens accounts for 3–4% of the volume of the eyeball.

2.2.2 *The Selection of Examination Order*

1. CT: It is the optimal method for this lesion, which may show the size and shape of eyeball whether normal or not.
2. MRI: It can be used to accurately measure the length of the eyeball, the size of the lens, and the thickness of the choroid and sclera to provide important information for clinical treatment.

2.2.3 *Imaging Performance*

1. CT performance: The eyeball and the orbital volume become smaller; the lens is larger with obtuse margin; the vitreum is normal; the extraocular muscles and optic nerve are slender (Fig. 2.3).
2. MRI performance: On the ipsilateral side of microphthalmia, the extraocular muscles are slender (Fig. 2.4). The optic nerve may be slender or absent. The subarachnoid space around the optic nerve becomes wider. The anterior atrium of the eyeball deepens when small eyeball is accompanied with concomitant glaucoma.

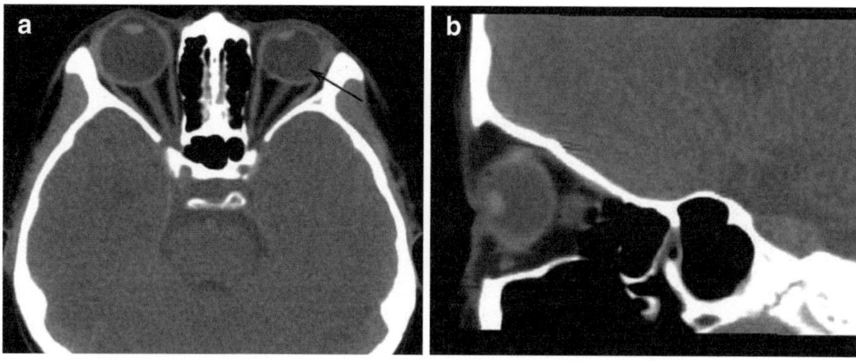

Fig. 2.3 Left simple microphthalmia. (**a**) Axial CT scan shows that the left eyeball is significantly smaller with normal shape; the lens is visible but moves forward; anterior atrium becomes shallow; the optic nerve and extraocular muscles are slender. (**b**) Sagittal CT scan shows that the left eyeball is smaller with normal shape; the lens moves forward; anterior atrium becomes shallow; the density of the vitreum is homogeneous

2.2.4 Evaluation

CT examination has unique advantages in the imaging of congenital microphthalmia as it is not affected by the opacity of the refractive media. Thus, it can clearly show the changes of the eyeball, internal cyst, optic nerve, ocular muscle, and orbital bone. It can not only identify the diagnosis and classification of microphthalmia, but also make accurate quantitative evaluation of the orbital volume, thus providing valuable information for the treatment of microphthalmia.

MRI is beneficial to more clearly observe other accompanying abnormalities, including some subtle lesions such as underdevelopment or detachment of the retina.

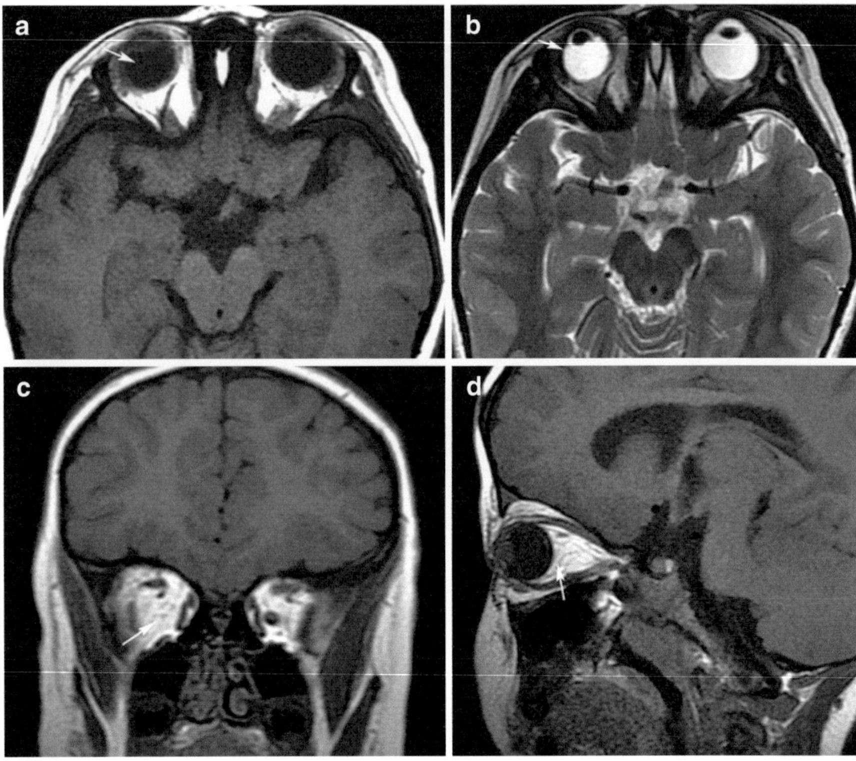

Fig. 2.4 Right simple microphthalmia. (**a**) Axial scan of T1WI shows that the right orbital cavity becomes smaller; the eyeball becomes significantly smaller with normal shape; the lens is visible but moves forward; the anterior atrium becomes shallow and the superior rectus is slender. (**b**) Axial scan of T2WI shows that the volume of the right eyeball becomes significantly smaller; the lens becomes larger in size and lower in signal and it moves anteriorly resulting in a shallower anterior atrium. (**c**) Coronal scan of T1WI shows that the right optic nerve is absent and the extraocular muscles are more slender compared with that of the contralateral side. (**d**) Sagittal scan of T1WI shows smaller right orbit cavity without normal optic nerve

2.3 Optic Disc Defect and Retrobulbar Cyst

Defective microphthalmia includes congenital microphthalmos with optic disc defect and cyst, and congenital microphthalmos with orbital cyst. An eyeball with small cyst and normal shape and size usually has partial function, while an underdeveloped eyeball with obvious defect and large cyst is nonfunctional. The shape of the eyeball may be normal or unable to retain. The lens may not develop or dislocate.

2.3.1 *Pathological Features*

With complete or partial defect of disc, usually accompanied by the defects of iris or choroid.

2.3.2 *Imaging Examination*

1. Ultrasonic: Optimal method for this lesion.
2. CT: It shows whether the shape or internal structure of the affected eyeball is normal, such as calcification.
3. MRI: It shows the lesion more clearly, which is helpful to differentiate from other lesions.

2.3.3 *Imaging Performance*

1. Ultrasound performance: Simple optic disc defect manifests as defected choroid sclera expanding back out with clear boundary and usually accompanied by the retinal detachment. Morning glory syndrome manifests as that the optic disc and the surrounding areas move back and sag. The posterior pole bulges with clear boundary. Irregular weak echo may be shown in the area of depression.
2. CT performance: Simple optic disc defect manifests as incomplete eye ring with defect at the connecting part of optic nerve and eyeball; elliptic or irregular cystic low-density area with clear boundary can be seen if a cyst is formed, which is connected or adjacent to incomplete eyeball, generally locating below the eyeball and behind the eyelid (Fig. 2.5). Morning glory syndrome manifests as a V bulges in the optic disc. The connection of the optic nerve and the eyeball is in expanding funnel shape and the depression is filled with hypo-dense tissue (Fei et al. 2013).
3. MRI performance: Retrobulbar cyst is hypo-intense on T1WI and hyper-intense on T2WI. When retinal detachment occurs, "V"-shape signal with iso-intense on T1WI and hyper-intense on T2WI can be seen at the posterior part of eyeball. Morning glory syndrome manifests as a funnel expansion area with iso-intense on T1WI and hyper-intense on T2WI (Fig. 2.6).

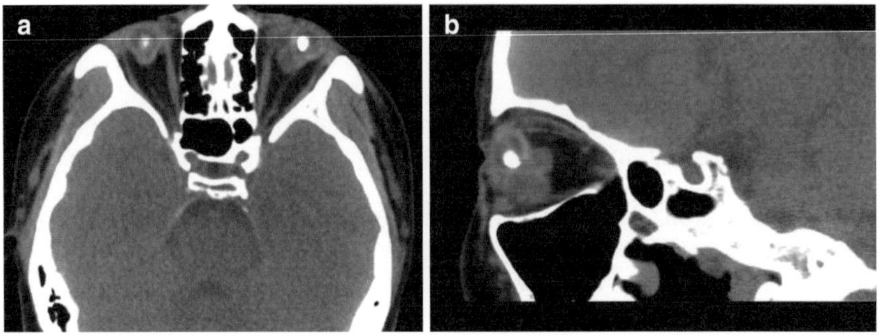

Fig. 2.5 Bilateral optic disc defect and posterior cyst of left eyeball. (**a**) The axial CT scan shows that the bilateral eyeballs become obviously small and flat; the lens becomes more hyper-dense and distorted; a cystic hunch can be seen behind the left eyeball. (**b**) The sagittal CT scan shows that the left eyeball is irregularly lobulated; the density of the lens increases and an oval cystic hunch can be seen at the posterior of the eyeball

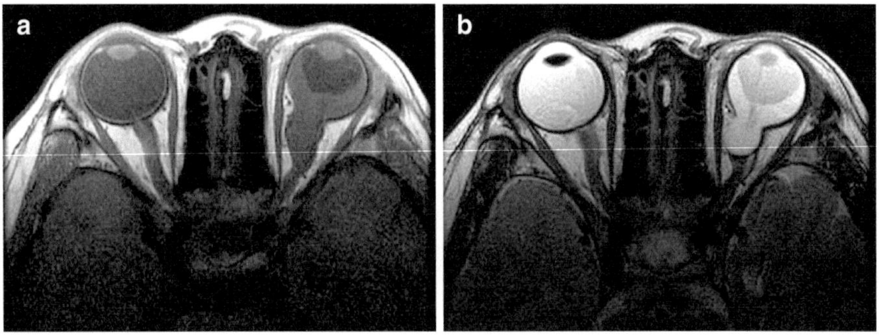

Fig. 2.6 Left optic disc defect and retrobulbar cyst. (**a**) The axial scan of T1W1 shows that the left eyeball becomes slightly smaller; the lens moves anteriorly. An iso-intense hunch can be seen at the optic disc of posterior of eyeball; and arc iso-intense signal can be seen at the posterior of eyeball. (**b**) The axial scan of T2W1 shows arc hyper-intensity at the posterior of the left eyeball and cystic hyper-intensity at the optic disc

2.3.4 Evaluation

CT may show the abnormal changes of the defected small eyeball and concomitant cyst, but some other lesions, such as congenital cystic eyeball, sclera staphyloma of posterior eyeball, dermoid cyst, cystic degeneration of optic nerve glioma, meningocele, and hemangioma, should be distinguished.

Congenital cystic eyeball means that the optic vesicle does not sag, resulting in one or more capsules being formed. Intraocular structures are usually absent while lens can be visible sometimes. Sclera staphyloma of posterior eyeball refers to any congenital or acquired focal expansion of eyeball wall. The expansion is not confined to the optic disc. The bulging part and the eyeball are at obtuse angle and the size of eyeball is usually normal.

MRI can show the abnormal signs of the orbit, which is useful to distinguish from other orbital lesions.

2.4 Permanent Primordial Vitreous Hyperplasia

2.4.1 Pathological Features

1. The mass behind the lens is composed of vascular loose connective tissues, including hyperplasia of fiber blood tissues and vitreous artery remnants.
2. The mass is connected forward with the posterior surface of the lens.
3. The vitreous artery covered by retina is connected backward with the optic disc.
4. Cartilage and bony tissues can be seen in the tumor.

2.4.2 Imaging Examination

1. CT: It is optimal for this lesion, which may show the lesion's location and shape as well as calcification.
2. MRI: It may show more detailed lesions and surrounding abnormalities, thus providing more information for differential diagnosis.

2.4.3 Imaging Performance

1. CT performance: The eyeball becomes smaller. Hyper-vascular original vitreous proliferations manifest as zonal or conical soft tissues between the lens and optic disc (Figs. 2.7 and 2.8a, b).
2. MRI performance: The signal of vitreum increases on both T1WI and T2WI. Tubular soft tissues with clear boundary are connected from posterior lens to front retinal optic disc. In addition, a triangle or "wine cup"-shaped or irregular mass behind the lens can be seen, which is iso- or slightly hypo-intense on both T1WI and T2WI. The vitreous artery and fibrous vessel membrane enhance, while the proliferated fibrous connective tissues do not (Fig. 2.8c, d).

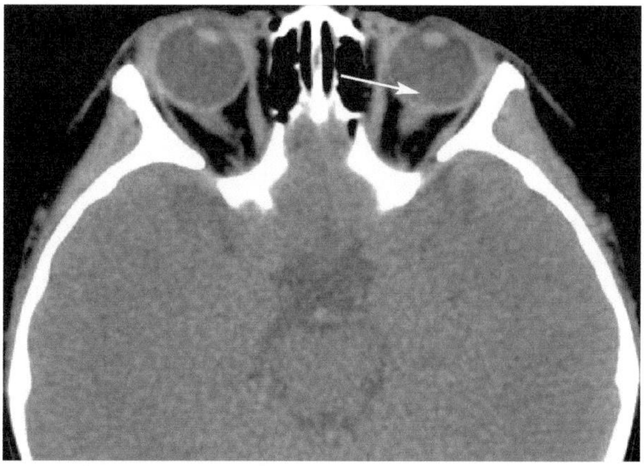

Fig. 2.7 Left permanent primordial vitreous hyperplasia. The axial scan of non-contrast CT shows slightly hyper-dense banded soft tissue posterior to left lens, connecting backward to the optic disc

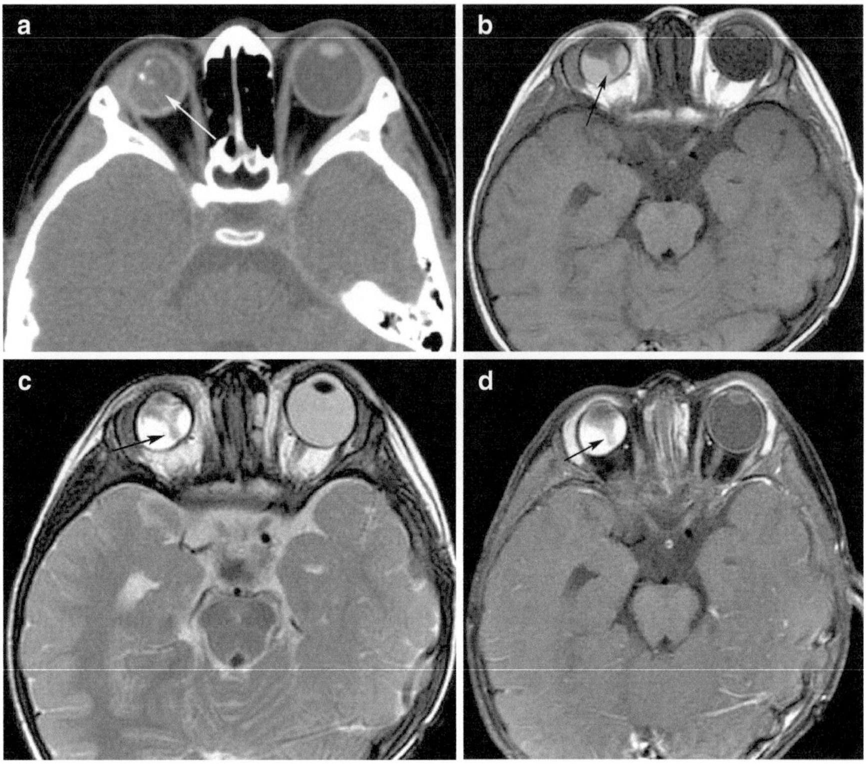

Fig. 2.8 Right permanent primordial vitreous hyperplasia. (**a**) The axial scan of non-contrast CT shows smaller eyeball and lens as well as shallow anterior chamber on the right side. In addition, banded soft tissue (*white arrow*) can be found to connect from posterior lens to the optic disc. (**b**) The axial scan of non-contrast T1W1 shows that right eyeball becomes smaller. Slight hypo-intense banded soft tissue (*black arrow*) in the hyper-intense vitreum can be found to connect from posterior lens to the optic disc. (**c**) The axial scan of T2W1 shows that slight hyper-intense banded soft tissue (*black arrow*) in the hyper-intense vitreum can be found to connect from posterior lens to the optic disc. (**d**) The axial scan of contrast fat-suppressing MRI shows that the banded soft tissue does not enhance

2.4.4 Evaluation

MRI has a higher sensitivity and specificity to show lesions in the eyeball with leukokoria than CT. CT and MRI both can show the shape of soft tissue in the vitreum clearly. CT is more sensitive for calcification, which is beneficial to distinguish from other lesions in eyeball. However, CT is not as sensitive as MRI in the assessment of detailed information in the lesion. Therefore, both CT and MRI are recommended to assess the lesion in the eyeball, if possible.

2.5 Coats Disease

The diagnostic criteria of coats disease is the idiopathic retinal capillary expansion, accompanied by infiltration of the retina and frequent exudative retinal detachment. The characteristics of this disease are as follows: male, school-aged children and juveniles, monocular lesions, no calcification, normal size of eyeball, and crescent-shaped hyper-dense soft tissue in the posterior eyeball. Patients with this disease mostly complain with decreased vision, strabismus, and white reflection in pupil area (Grosso et al. 2015).

2.5.1 Pathological Features

1. Retinal lipid exudation in the early period.
2. Lots of protein effusion and bleeding with part or entire detachment of retina in the middle period.
3. The exudation replaced by connective tissue in the late period, accompanied by inflammation or atrophy of the eyeball.

2.5.2 Imaging Examination

1. Ultrasound: It is the optimal examination for this disease.
2. CT: It may identify whether calcification occurs or not.
3. MRI: It is helpful to distinguish from other lesions as it may show more detailed characteristics of the lesion.

2.5.3 Imaging Performance

1. Ultrasound: The retina with lesion thickens irregularly. The sub-retinal fluids may present as transparent, cloudy, or uneven dots because of different contents. The retinal detachment refers to V- or Y-type light band.
2. CT performance: The lesion confines to the retina, presenting as thickening of retina. The exudations are located below the retina leading to the retinal detachment. The exudation presents as well-defined hyper-density if with lots of protein or accompanied by bleeding. Slight enhancement of retina can be seen.
3. MRI performance: It may show retinal detachment, bleeding, and leakage more clearly. The shape of sub-retinal effusion varies greatly, which may be half-moon, lenticular, or strip shape. The signal is associated with the protein amount in the exudation. The lesion is hyper-intense on T1WI and iso- or hyper-intense

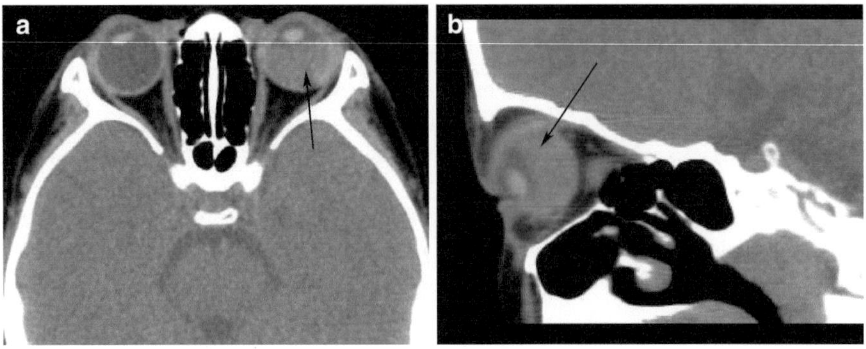

Fig. 2.9 Coats disease. (**a**) The axial scan of non-contrast CT shows slight hyper-density with "half-moon" shape in the posterior vitreum behind the lens of left eyeball. (**b**) The sagittal scan of non-contrast CT shows slight hyper-density in the posterior vitreum, the anterior of which is clear to the lens

on T2WI if with high-level protein. The lesion is hypo-intense on T1WI and hyper-intense on T2WI if with low-level protein. If bleeding occurs, the signal is different due to the time of bleeding. No enhancement can be seen for this lesion (Fig. 2.9).

2.5.4 *Evaluation*

Ultrasonic examination is flexible, convenient, and nontraumatic and it may be performed again and again. The fundus fluorescein angiography, indirect ophthalmoscope, and cytological analysis of retinal exudations are the main basis for diagnosis. CT is optimal to assess whether calcification exists or not while MRI is more sensitive to show retinal exudation, detachment, and hemorrhage. Contrast scanning is beneficial to distinguish from neuroblastoma. In addition, MRI plays an important role in comprehensive display of the scope, nature, and stage of the lesions.

2.6 Dermoid Cyst and Epidermoid Cyst

Dermoid cyst and epidermoid cyst are mostly seen in sphenoid bone suture, zygomatic, and winglet of adolescents. The mass is cystic, well defined, with slightly wave motion, with no tenderness, presenting as partial bulge, with normal eyeball.

2.6.1 *Pathological Features*

1. The wall of epidermoid cyst only has epidermal tissue, including basal cell stratum of squamous epithelium, spine cell layer, stratum corneum, and fibrous tissue layer. The contents of the cyst are epidermal keratinocytes.
2. Apart from the squamous epithelial layers, the dermoid cyst also contains squamous epithelial layers, sebaceous glands, sweat glands, etc.

2.6.2 *Imaging Examination*

1. B ultrasound: It may show various acoustic properties in the cyst but it is difficult to make qualitative and positioning diagnosis.
2. CT: It is beneficial to locate the lesion and it may show the normal structure of the orbit. According to the shape, low density of the contents, and close relationship with bone and joint, the nature of the lesion can be assessed preliminarily.
3. MRI: The resolution of soft tissue is higher to show the involvement of soft tissue around the lesions.

2.6.3 *Imaging Performance*

1. B ultrasound: The signal of orbital cyst varies due to different contents. The cyst shows mixed high echo if with mixed fluid and keratinization. The cyst shows high echo surrounded by fluid dark if keratinization is surrounded by fluid in the cyst. The cyst shows homogeneous hypoecho if just with fluid. The acoustic attenuation is not obvious and the echo of anterior wall is higher than that of posterior wall.
2. CT performance: Cysts are mostly located near the suture of sphenoid bone's greater wing and lesser wing or zygomatic frontal suture, manifesting as oval, round, or dumbbell shape. Epidermoid cyst may be shown as homogeneous density of fluid or soft tissue (Fig. 2.10a). Dermoid cyst be shown as fatty density (Fig. 2.11a–c) or mixed high and low density. No enhancement can be seen in

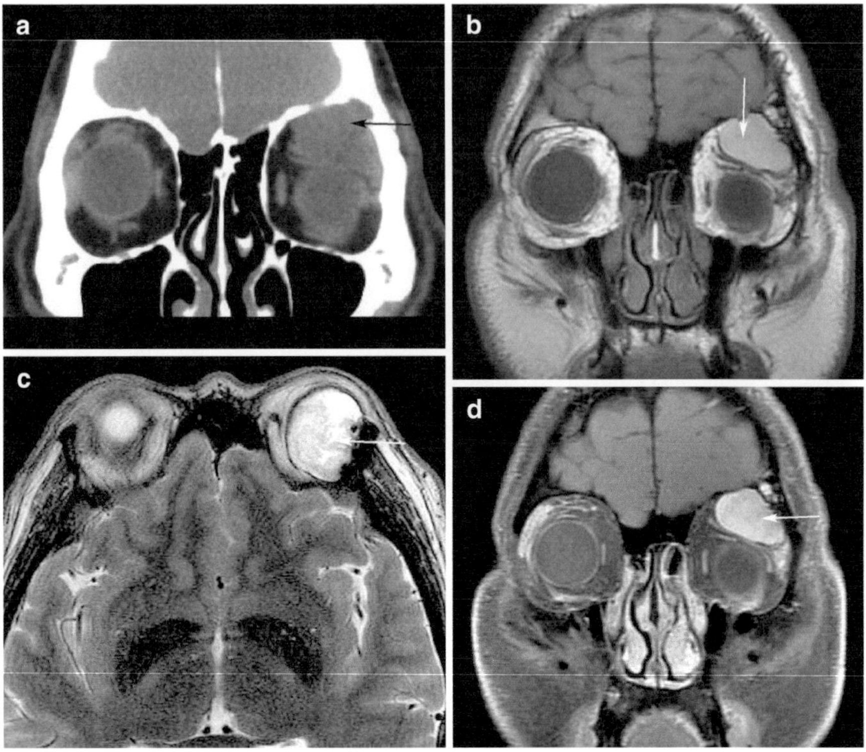

Fig. 2.10 Left epidermoid cyst. (**a**) The coronal scan of non-contrast CT shows that semielliptical soft tissue (*black arrow*) can be seen in extra-muscular cone space of the superior lateral quadrant. The adjacent structures are depressed and displaced. The orbital suture widens. (**b**) The coronal scan of non-contrast T1WI shows that the lesion is hyper-intense and well defined. The lateral rectus muscle and supraocular muscle group are compressed and displaced. The eyeball moves down with normal shape. (**c**) The axial scan of T2WI shows that an oval heterogeneous hyper-intensity (*white arrow*) and patchy iso-intensity within can be seen in the superior lateral quadrant. (**d**) The coronal scan of contrast MRI with fat sat shows no enhancement of the lesion

both lesions while the cystic wall can be seen with moderate enhancement. Bony depression or aperture can be seen around the cyst.

3. MRI performance: The walls of dermoid and epidermoid cysts show slightly hypo-intense on both T1WI and T2WI. Dermoid cyst mostly shows homogeneous hypo-intense on T1WI and hyper-intense on T2WI. Sometimes, dermoid cyst shows homo- or heterogeneous hyper-intense on both T1WI and T2WI. No enhancement can be seen in the lesion while the cystic wall can be seen with slightly enhancement (Fig. 2.10d). The signal of dermoid cyst is complicated. It will be hyper-intense on both T1WI and T2WI if with sweat and sebum (Fig. 2.12a,b). It will be mixed hyper-, moderate, and hypo-intense if with lots of debris and hair. No enhancement can be seen (Fig. 2.12c).

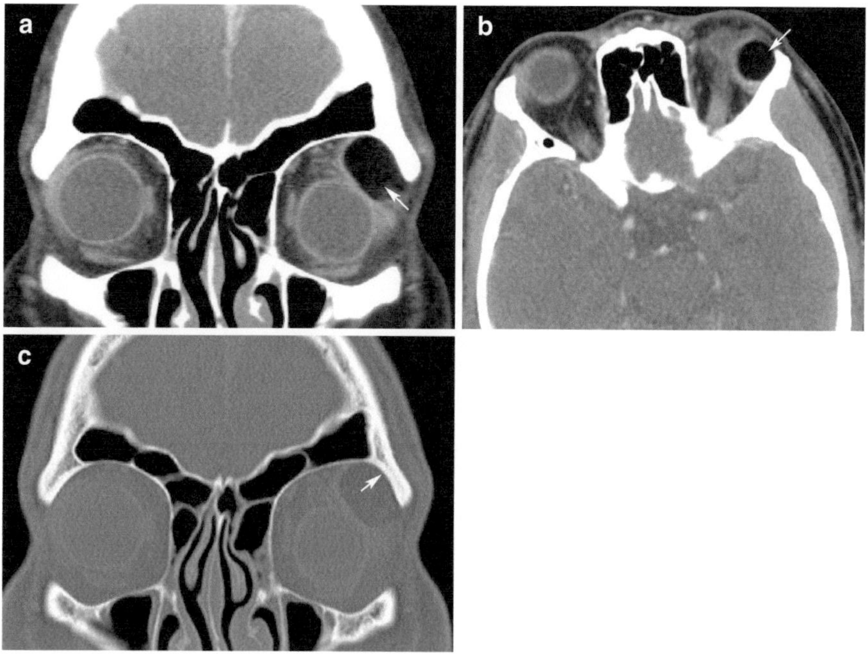

Fig. 2.11 Left dermoid cyst (CT). (**a**) The coronal scan of contrast CT shows that a semielliptical mass (*white arrow*) with CT value of -65HU can be seen in extra-muscular cone space of the superior lateral quadrant. Adjacent lateral rectus muscle and supra-ocular muscle group are compressed and displaced. (**b**) The axial scan of contrast CT shows that the lesion (*white arrow*) is well defined but has close relationship with lacrimal gland. (**c**) The coronal scan of CT reformatted with bone window shows that adjacent bony wall (*white arrow*) is depressed and the bony edge is smooth

2.6.4 Evaluation

Ultrasound cannot show the whole of the cyst but just a part. It is good at indirectly reflecting the histological structure according to the echo. Meanwhile, it may make hemodynamic assessment of the cyst, such as compressibility. Because dermoid cyst varies greatly in range (from intraorbital to extraorbtial) and density (from negative to bony density), CT is considered as the optimal examination for this lesion. MRI may show the intensity formed by mixed contents and the relationship with other surrounding structures. It has the highest accuracy of localization and positioning of all imaging examinations, providing great significance for this lesion.

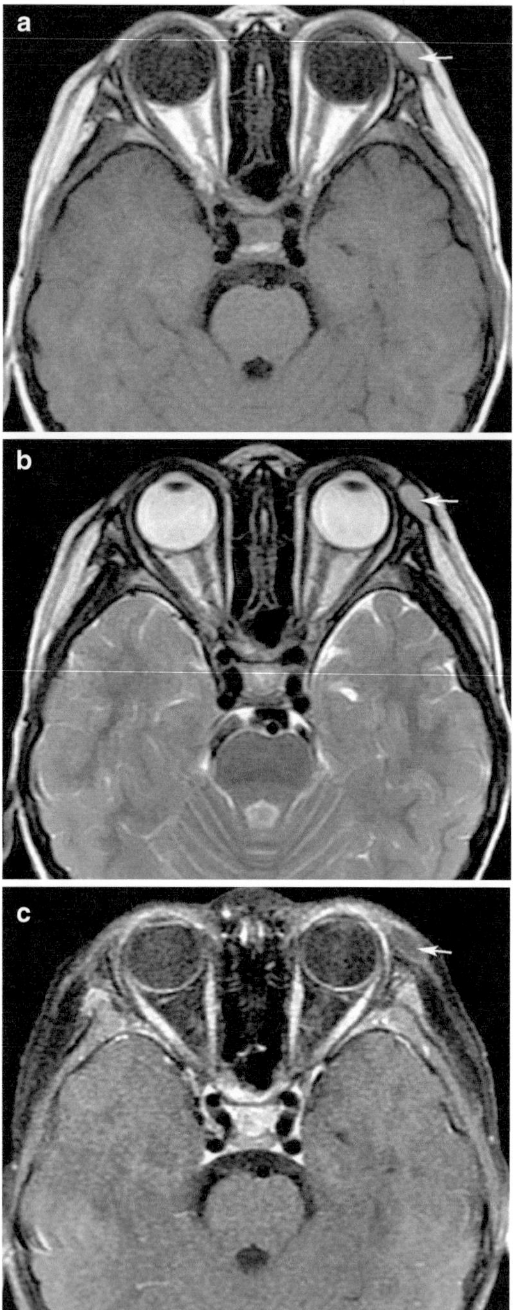

Fig. 2.12 Left dermoid cyst (MRI). (**a**) The axial scan of T1WI shows an elliptical lesion that is slightly hyper-intense in the temporal subcutaneous tissue of left orbit (*white arrow*). (**b**) The axial scan of T2WI shows that the lesion is hyper-intense. (**c**) The axial scan of contrast T1WI with fat suppression shows the signal of the lesion decreased and without enhancement. The wall enhances slightly

2.7 Langerhans' Cell Histiocytosis

2.7.1 Pathological Features

1. The cell has medium size and unclear margin. The cytoplasm may be clear or eosinophilic. The nucleus may be oval or irregular usually with visible notch, and characteristic nuclear groove can be seen in nest, tufted, or diffuse distribution.
2. This lesion is often accompanied by a large number of eosinophils, lymphocytes, neutrophils, and plasma cells.
3. Tumor cells have strong expression of CD1a and S2100 protein in immunohistochemistry; different expressions of CD68, Syn, and Ki67 3–25%; and no expression of CD20, CD3, CD30, MPO, EMA, and CD21 (Yongjae 2009).

2.7.2 Imaging Examination

1. CT: This lesion's diagnosis mostly depends on the changes of the involved bone, which can be clearly and accurately shown using CT. Thus, CT is the most important imaging examination for this lesion.
2. MRI: The resolution of soft tissue is better when using MR than CT, which makes MR more accurate to show the mass's size, involving range and relationship with adjacent structures. Especially, it is more reliable in the manifestation of the brain parenchyma, brain meninges, optic nerve, extraocular muscles, bone marrow, and other structures than CT. Thus, it is the most important imaging examination for the surgical treatment and evaluation of prognosis.

2.7.3 Imaging Performance

1. CT performance: This lesion mostly occurs at the conjunction of orbit's upper and lateral walls. Osteolytic destruction is mostly seen, with large bone defects formed. The residual edge is irregular but clear with no sclerosis (Figs. 2.13a and 2.14a). Soft-tissue mass with heterogeneous density can be seen at the corresponding portion. Pieces of bones or small dead bones can be seen sometimes. The lesion can be seen with moderate to strong enhancement.
2. MRI performance: Irregular soft-tissue mass can be seen at the corresponding portion of bone defect area, which is mostly slightly hypo-intense on T1WI (Figs. 2.13b and 2.14b) and iso- or hyper-intense on T2WI (Figs. 2.13c and 2.14c). Some structures are depressed and displaced. Adjacent subcutaneous tissue of frontal, temporal scalp, temporalis, and meninges thickens if involved, with moderate to strong enhancement (Figs. 2.13d and 2.14d).

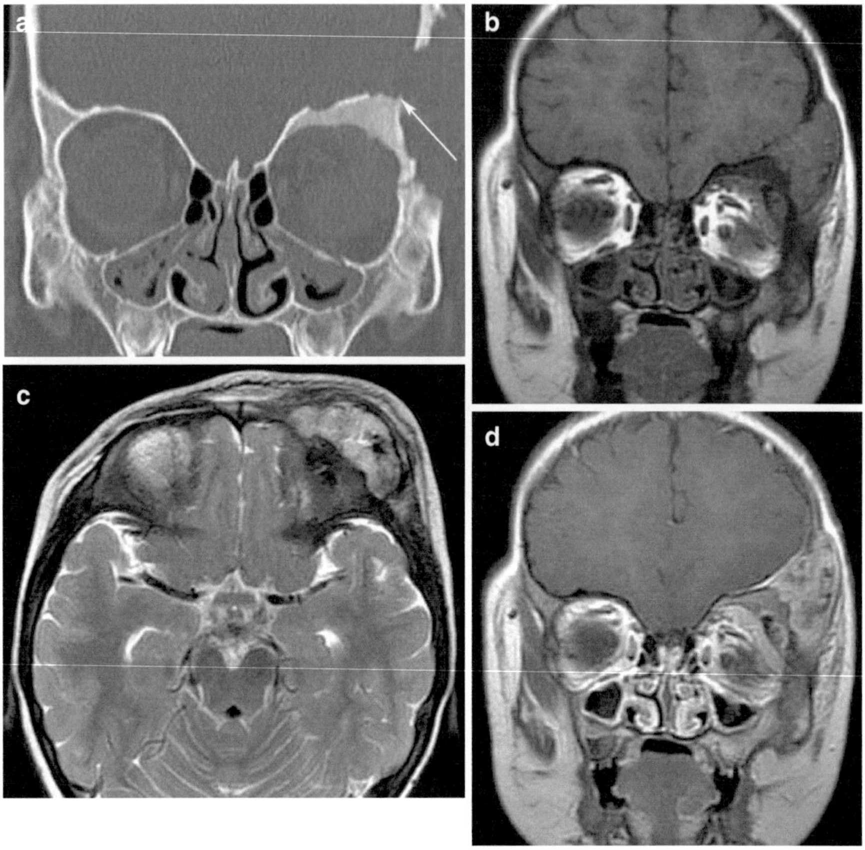

Fig. 2.13 Left Langerhans' cell histiocytosis. (**a**) The coronal scan of non-contrast CT reformatted with bone window shows local bony defect in the left frontal bone. The margin is irregular but smooth (*white arrow*). (**b**) The coronal scan of T1WI shows that an iso-intense mass can be seen in the left frontal bone where bony defect formed. The extra-muscular cone space in the superior lateral quadrant is involved, in which some structures are depressed and displaced. (**c**) The axial scan of T2WI shows that a mixed hyper- and hypo-intense mass can be seen in the portion where bony defect is formed in left frontal-sphenoid greater wing. (**d**) The coronal scan of contrast T1WI shows heterogeneous and strong enhancement of the mass. The left frontal meninges are thickening and enhanced

2.7.4 Evaluation

This disease is commonly seen in teenagers under 20 years old. If the bony defect is obvious while the patients just present as exophthalmos, minor inflammatory changes, or other slightly symptoms; in other words, if the bone changes do not correspond with the clinical symptoms, then Langerhans' cell hyperplasia should be considered. The combination of CT and MRI plays a greater role in the diagnosis and treatment of this disease (Nicollas et al. 2010).

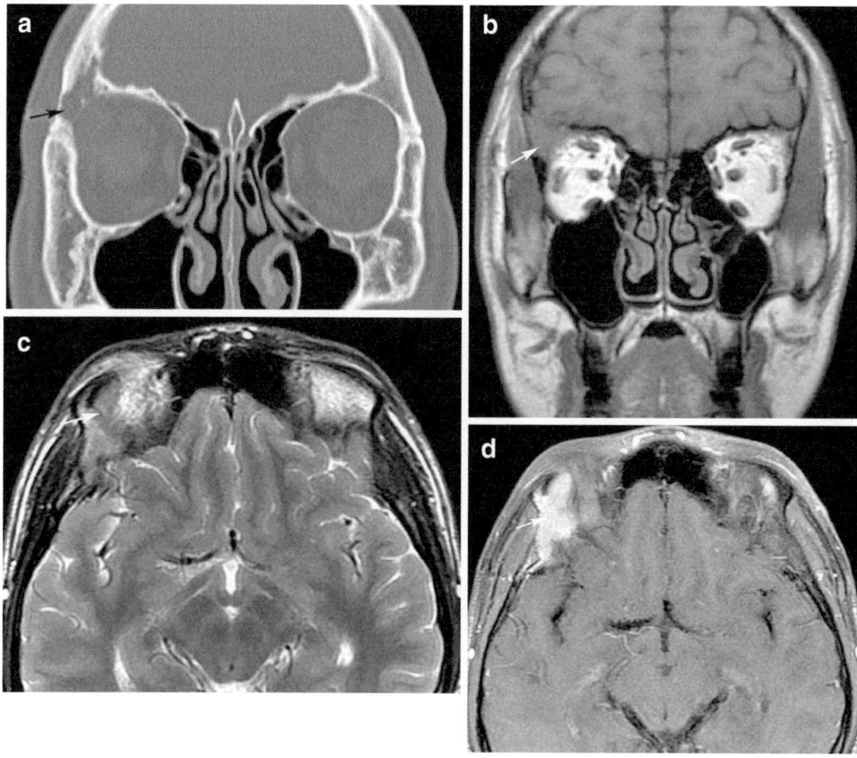

Fig. 2.14 Right Langerhans' cell histiocytosis. (**a**) The coronal scan of CT reformatted with bone window shows local bony defect in the lateral-superior wall of the right orbit. The margin is irregular but smooth (*black arrow*). (**b**) The coronal scan of T1WI shows that an iso-intense mass can be seen in the right frontal bone where bony defect formed. The extra-muscular cone space in the superior lateral quadrant is involved. (**c**) The axial scan of T2WI shows an iso-intense mass in the portion where bony defect is formed in right frontal-sphenoid greater wing. (**d**) The axial scan of contrast T1WI with fat suppression shows homogeneous and strong enhancement of the mass. The adjacent frontal meninges are thickening and enhanced

2.8 Neurofibromatosis

Neurofibromatosis (NF) is divided into two types and type I is usually with orbital-facial involvement. The characteristics of orbital-facial involvement of NF-I are introduced as follows.

2.8.1 *Pathological Features*

1. The neurofibroma in the orbit is divided into three types: plexiform neurofibroma, diffuse neurofibroma, and confined neurofibroma. Neurofibroma originated from peripheral nerves has no capsule. The plexiform neurofibroma is mostly seen with orbital involvement.
2. The confined neurofibroma usually has pseudo-capsule, with shuttle-shaped cell bundle and collagen fiber bundle in stroma. In addition, certain amount of collagen can be found in the stroma.
3. The plexiform neurofibroma can be seen with proliferated nerve sheath cells, axons, and fiber cell wrap in the mucous matrix. The intratumoral vessels are significantly increased.
4. The diffuse neurofibroma can be seen with proliferated nerve sheath cells, axons, and nerve fiber cell wrap, without obvious nerve sheath.
5. Most of the lesions are solid with moderate collagen. Some lesions are mucus, represented as jelly sample (Jackson et al. 1993; Anderson and Gutmann 2015).

2.8.2 *Imaging Examination*

1. CT: It is recommended as the optimal method as it may show the abnormalities of bones and soft tissues, especially the former one.
2. MRI: It may show the involvement range and accompanied intracranial tumors clearly.

2.8.3 *Imaging Performance*

1. CT performance: The orbital bone dysplasia usually presents as bony defect of sphenoid greater and smaller wings, oval enlarged orbit (Fig. 2.15a), and obviously enlarged middle cranial fossa (Fig. 2.15b). Meningocele or meningoencephalocele with exophthalmos may occur when orbital defect is very serious. The plexiform neurofibroma manifests as ill-defined, irregular, and invasive mass, accompanied by changes such as thickened temporalis and eyelids, and irregular thickened extraocular muscles. The lesion may be extended to all adjacent structures in the orbit, such as the lacrimal glands, fat, and extraocular muscles. Periorbital area such as soft tissues in temporal fossa and frontal part can also be involved (Fig. 2.15, Fig. 2.16). Other accompanied tumors in the orbit

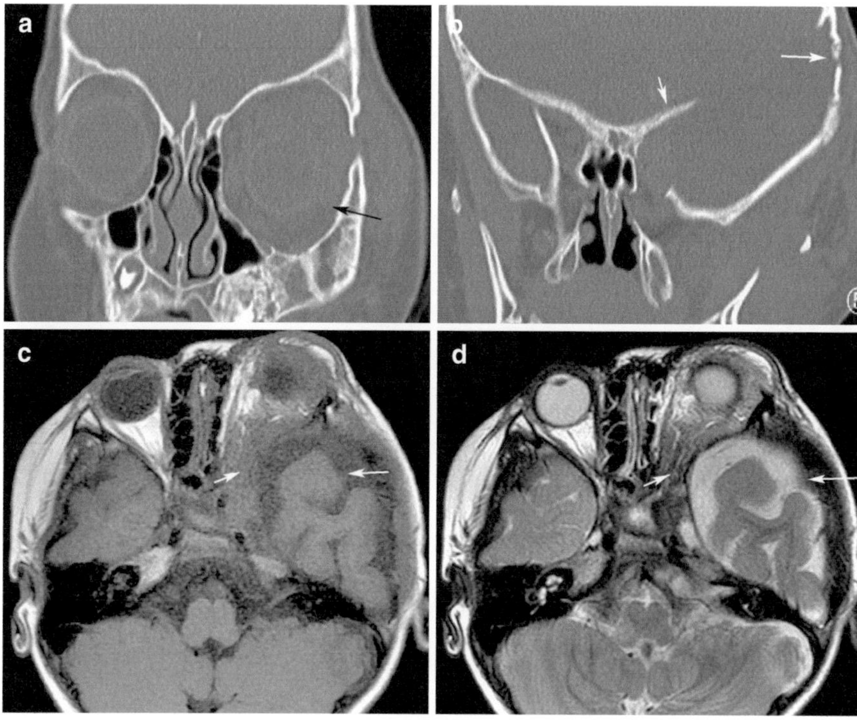

Fig. 2.15 Type I of neurofibromatosis. (**a**) The coronal scan of CT reformatted with bone window shows obvious enlargement of left orbit with a "vertical oval" shape. (**b**) The coronal scan of CT reformatted with bone window shows dysplasia of sphenoid greater and smaller wing (*short arrow*). The superior orbital fissure and the left temporal-squamosal fissure (*long arrow*) are obviously enlarged and sclerotic. The adjacent bone sclerosis is visible. (**c**) The axial scan of T1WI shows the iso-intense, ill-defined, and irregular soft tissues in the left orbit, which partially wraps the temporal eyeball. In addition, the lesion extends to cavernous sinus through the widened superior orbital fissure. The shape of left temporal lobe is irregular (*long arrow*). (**d**) The axial scan of T2WI shows iso-intense soft tissues in the left orbit. The lacrimal gland is involved and widened obviously, presenting with slightly hyper-intense. The left middle cranial fossa is significantly expanded with temporal lobe dysplasia

include optic nerve gliomas, meningiomas, and schwannomas. The hydrops in the eyeball may result in giant eyeball.

2. MRI: CT is better to show the bony abnormalities of plexiform neurofibroma while MRI is better to show adjacent involvement. The plexiform or diffuse neurofibroma presents as ill-defined mass in the orbit with frontal-temporal subcutaneous tissues involved. The lesion extends backwards to the orbital apex; it invades cavernous sinus through the superior orbital fissure and pterygopalatine fossa and infratemporal fossa through the inferior orbital fissure. Nodular soft tissues can be seen in the orbit, with iso-intense on T1W1 (Figs. 2.15c and 2.16b) and iso- or slightly hyper-intense on T2WI (Figs. 2.15d and 2.16c). Sometimes, "target sign" can be seen in teenagers' orbit and temporal fossa, with medium-strong enhancement. Contrast T1WI with fat suppression is optimal to show the sign (Fig. 2.16d).

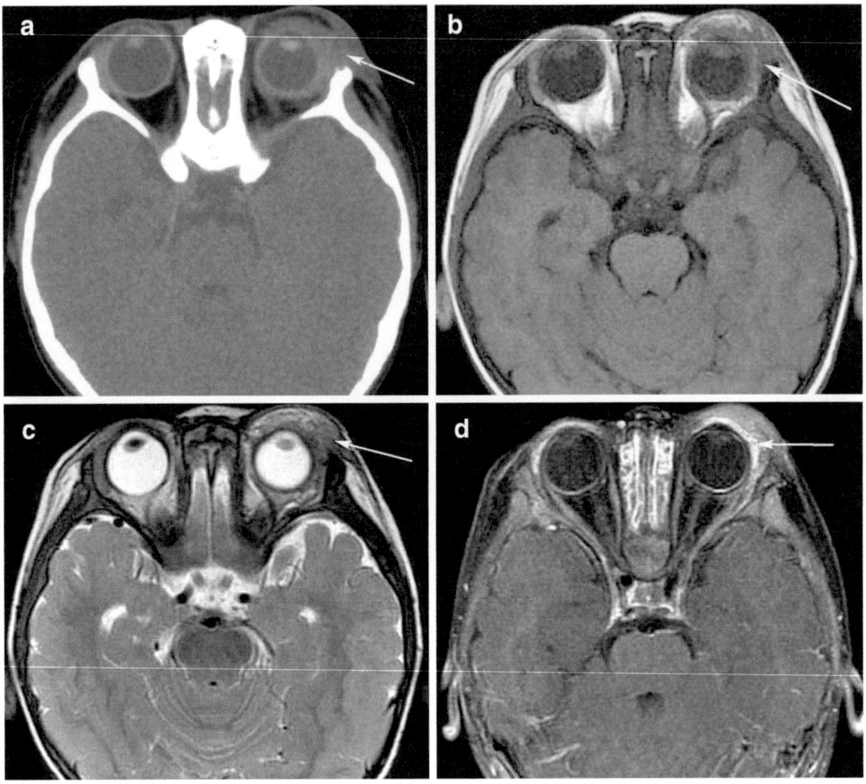

Fig. 2.16 Type I of neurofibromatosis. (**a**) The axial scan of non-contrast CT shows irregular soft-tissue mass (*white arrow*) at the temporal side of the left eyeball, which partially wraps the eyeball. The left superior orbital fissure is widened and the sphenoid wing becomes shorter. (**b**) The axial scan of T1WI shows iso-intense soft tissues at the temporal side of left eyeball (*white arrow*), which is not clearly divided with lacrimal gland. (**c**) The axial scan of T2WI shows that the signal of the lesion is heterogeneous and slightly hyper-intense. (**d**) The contrast scan with fat suppression shows the mass with heterogeneous and medium enhancement

2.8.4 Evaluation

Although cheap and feasible, X-ray just shows the abnormal changes in the orbit indirectly. Ultrasound makes little sense to the qualitative diagnosis and it is difficult to show the lesion's extent completely. Multi-slice spiral CT may show the bony abnormalities and the extended range of the lesions in the orbit. In addition, it may be used to assess whether cavernous sinus or pterygopalatine fossa is involved according to the shape and density. However, it is difficult to show the relationships with surrounding structures and whether intracranial accompanied tumor exists or not. MRI may show the extent of the lesion, and its relationships with surrounding structures and concurrent tumors in other locations. However, it is difficult to clearly show the bony abnormalities. The diagnostic standard of NF-I is complicated and it needs to be combined with clinic. If both sphenoid dysplasia and plexiform neurofibroma are found, this disease should be diagnosed.

2.9 Fibrous Dysplasia

2.9.1 Pathological Features

1. Normal bone is replaced by the abnormal hyperplastic fibrous tissue.
2. The fibrous tissue includes hyperplastic fibroblasts, collagen fiber bundles, and swirling and weaving.
3. Marginal trabecula of the lesion is migrated with normal trabecula.

2.9.2 Imaging Examination

1. CT: It is the optimal examination to show the bony abnormalities as well as the lesion's extent and margin.
2. MRI: It is better to show soft tissue's changes than CT. It may clearly show the depression and displacement of intra- and extra-orbital structures, as well as whether the signal of soft tissue is normal or not.

2.9.3 Imaging Performance

1. CT performance: The affected bones are usually enlarged and the density of marrow cavity may be increased or decreased, homogeneous or heterogeneous. The lesion extends along the bone growing direction and it has no clear boundary with normal bone tissue. There is no periosteal reaction or soft-tissue mass. According to the lesion's density, it can be divided into three types: ground glass type, loofah type, and sclerotic type. The former two types are more common while the third type is just rarely seen among middle-aged or old patients. Ground glass type is defined that the lesion includes more fibrous component but less bony component with evenly distribution. Sclerotic type is defined that the lesion includes less fibrous component but more bony component with evenly distribution. The loofah type is defined that the lesion is composed of heterogeneously distributed fibrous and bony tissues, presenting as mixed hyper- and hypodensity. Pathologically, hyper-dense area means abnormal bony tissue based and hypo-dense area means fibrous tissue based (Fig. 2.17) (Lisle et al. 2008).
2. MRI performance: The lesion is mostly shown with hetero- or homogeneous hypo-intense on both T1WI and T2WI (mixed signals with a majority of low signals). The intensity and enhancement are different due to different fibrous, bony components in different areas. The lesion will be hypo-intense on T1WI and hyper-intense on T2WI if liquefaction and necrosis occur in the lesion. The lesion will be hyper-intense on T1WI if bleeding occurs. The residual bone marrow is also hyper-intense on T1WI. Fat suppression is helpful for the identification of hyper-intensity on T1WI.

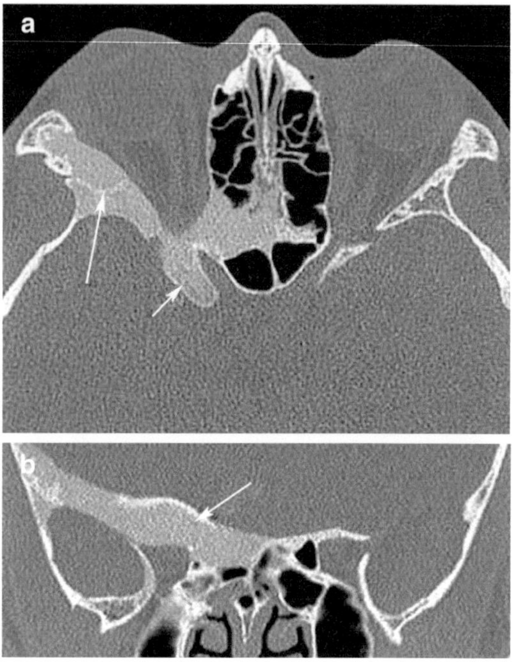

Fig. 2.17 Fibrous dysplasia. (**a**) The axial scan of CT reformatted with bone window shows that the right orbital wall, greater wing of sphenoid, smaller wing of sphenoid, and part of ethmoid bone are thickened with ground glass density (white arrow). (**b**) The coronal scan of CT reformatted with bone window shows that right smaller wing of sphenoid, sphenoid platform, and sphenoid body are thickened with ground glass density. The volume of the right orbital apex is smaller compared to that of the contralateral side

2.9.4 Evaluation

CT can clearly show the detail, margin, and affected extent of the cranial fibrous dysplasia, especially for the involvement of orbit, sinuses, and middle ear. In addition, it may identify the involvement of cranial channels such as optic canal, rotundum foramen, canalis pterygoid, oval foramen, superior orbital fissure, and inferior orbital fissure. Although bony change shown on MRI is not as good as CT, MRI has high sensitivity and resolution to show the lesion and soft tissue around more clearly, which has an important value on the evaluation of lesion's extent, complications, malignant, treatment choice, and evaluating the postoperative changes of the lesions and surrounding structures. Therefore, it serves as a supplementary examination of CT.

2.10 Crouzon Syndrome

Crouzon syndrome is also called craniofacial bone hypoplasia, which is an autosomal dominant genetic disease.

2.10.1 *Pathological Features*

1. The cranial sutures are closed earlier but the hand and foot are normal.
2. The ocular damage is caused by the earlier closing of cranial sutures, which leads to the intracranial hypertension, nerve traction, and coarctation of the optic nerve et al., resulting in the papilledema and optic nerve atrophy.

2.10.2 *Imaging Examination*

1. CT: It is the optimal examination as it may show the bony abnormalities of cranio-facial-orbital areas.
2. MRI: It may show the secondary changes of the intraocular structures, including the eyeball, optic nerve, and extraocular muscles. It may be used to show the development of brain, providing more evidence for the clinical assessment of the disease.
3. X-ray: If CT and MRI cannot be performed, the anteroposterior and lateral position films of the skull may show the preliminary skull malformation.

2.10.3 *Imaging Performance*

1. CT and MRI performance of the orbit: The orbit cavity becomes shallow. The greater wing of sphenoid is slim and moves forward and outside. The angle formed by the bilateral lateral wall is enlarged. The orbital apex is depressed sharper while the volume becomes smaller (Fig. 2.18a). The eyeball is depressed resulting in exophthalmos with normal shape and density. The optic nerve courses circuitously (Fig. 2.18b). The shape and location of extraocular muscles are abnormal. MRI may show the widened subarachnoid space around the optic nerve if optic atrophy occurs, which is hypo-intense on T1WI and hyper-intense on T2WI.
2. Other related abnormalities: Other related abnormalities include skull malformation, nonprogressive ventricle enlargement, maxillary bone dysplasia, and crossbite of upper and lower teeth. Chronic tonsillar hernia or Chiari I malformation may also be seen in some cases (Fig. 2.19). Nasal malformation includes

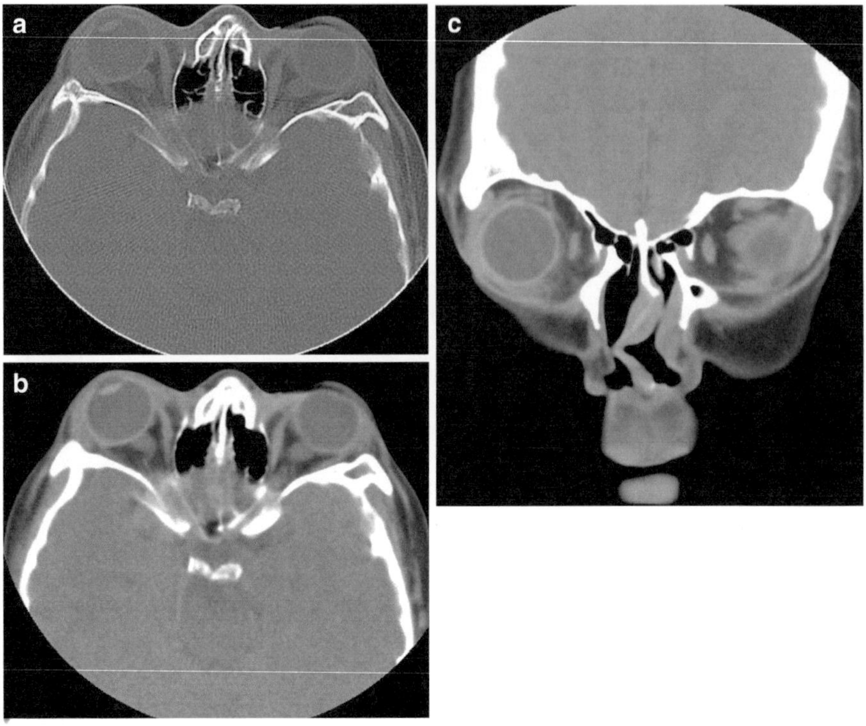

Fig. 2.18 Crouzon syndrome. (**a**) The axial scan of CT reformatted with bone window shows that the bilateral orbital cavities become shallow. The sphenoid greater wing becomes slender and moves forward and outside. The angle formed by the bilateral lateral wall is enlarged. (**b**) The axial scan of CT reformatted with soft-tissue window shows bilateral exophthalmos with normal shape and density of eyeball. The optic nerve courses circuitously. (**c**) The coronal scan of CT reformatted with soft-tissue window shows obvious deviation of nasal septum. The impression of skull plate becomes deepened and wavy

deviation of nasal septum (Fig. 2.18c), and stenosis or atresia of postnaris and nasopharyngeal cavity (Alexiou and Prodromou 2010).

3. X-ray performance: Lots of cranial malformations are caused by earlier closure of the skull sutures. The skull becomes thinner and the impressions increase and deepen in faveolate shape. The maxilla becomes smaller with deciduous teeth. The mandible protrusion can be seen. The orbital cavity becomes shallow and the optic nerve becomes smaller. The nasopharyngeal cavity becomes narrower; the skull base sags and the middle-posterior fossa deepen.

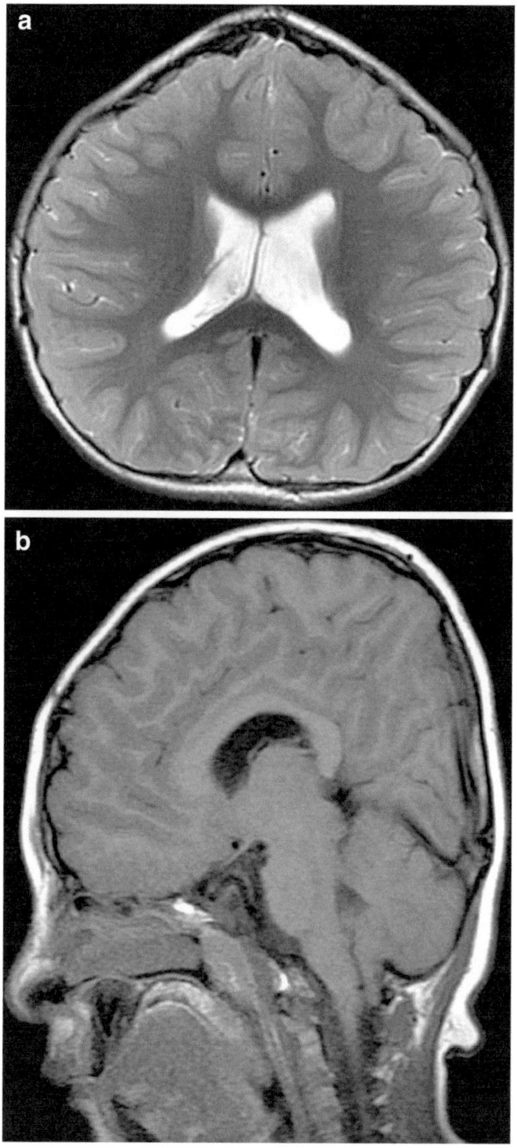

Fig. 2.19 Crouzon syndrome. (**a**) The axial scan of T2WI shows abnormal frontal bone and bilateral dilated ventricles. (**b**) The sagittal scan of T1WI shows deepened middle and posterior cranial fossa. The inferior margin of the cerebellar tonsil becomes sharp and herniates downward forming cerebellar herniation

2.10.4 Evaluation

CT may show the development of the craniofacial bone of the Crouzon syndrome and can provide three-dimensional reconstruction images, providing objective basis for clinical diagnosis and treatment. MRI may show the secondary changes of the eyeball, optic nerve, and extraocular muscles caused by orbital cavity narrowing. It may also show the parenchymal situation. MRI is a supplementary inspection method of CT as it plays an essential part in determining the lesion's degree and identifying treatment.

References

Alexiou GA, Prodromou N. Dandy-Walker malformation in Crouzon syndrome. J Child Neurol. 2010;25(5):653.

Anderson JL, Gutmann DH. Neurofibromatosis type 1. Handb Clin Neurol. 2015;132:75–86.

Davies DL. Anophthalmiaand microphthalmia. Orphanet J Rare Dis. 2007;2(1):501–2.

Fei P, Zhang Q, Zhao P, et al. Clinical characteristics and treatment of 22 eyes of morning glory syndrome associated with persistent hyperplastic primary vitreous. Br J Ophthalmol. 2013;97(10):1262–7.

Grosso A, Pellegrini M, Cereda MG, et al. Pearls and pitfalls in diagnosis and management of coats disease. Retina. 2015;35(4):614–23.

Jackson IT, Carbonnel A, Potparic Z, et al. Orbitotemporal neurofibromatosis: classification and treatment. Plast Reconstr Surg. 1993;92(1):1–11.

Lisle DA, Paj M, Maskiell CD. Imaging of craniofacial fibrous dysplasia. J Med Imaging Radiat Oncol. 2008;52(4):325–32.

Nicollas R, Belaich H, Roman S, et al. Head and neck manifestation and prognosis of Langerhans' cell histiocytosis in children. Int J Pediatr Otorhinolaryngol. 2010;74(6):669–73.

Yongjae LAF. Orbital Langerhans cell Histiocytosis. Int Ophthalmol Clin. 2009;49(1):123–31.

Chapter 3
Ocular Trauma

Han Lv, Zhenchang Wang, and Zhengyu Zhang

3.1 Eyeball Injury

3.1.1 Pathological Features

1. Eyeball damage, including hyphema, traumatic cataract, dislocation and rupture of the crystalline lens, vitreous hemorrhage, retinal and choroidal detachment, ocular rupture, and intraocular foreign body.
2. It can induce necrosis of the tissue, blood vessel reaction, tissue tearing, and displacement.
3. Penetrating wounds of the eye are based on the trajectory of the sharp weapon.

3.1.2 Order of the Imaging Examination

1. CT scan: CT scan is the first choice. It can reveal the altered shape and density with high resolution and speed.
2. MRI scans: Patients with simple eyeball injury usually do not need MRI scan. MRI is applicable when optic nerve or extraocular muscle injuries are suspected. Metal foreign bodies are contraindications.

H. Lv • Z. Wang (✉)
Department of Radiology, Beijing Friendship Hospital, Capital Medical University, Beijing, China
e-mail: cjr.wzhch@vip.163.com

Z. Zhang
Department of Radiology, Beijing Unicare ENT Hospital, Beijing, China

Z. Wang et al. (eds.), *Diagnostic Imaging of Ophthalmology*,
https://doi.org/10.1007/978-94-024-1060-0_3

3.1.3 Radiologic Features

1. CT scan: It usually includes (1) volume change of the eye ball (increase or decrease), due to hemorrhage or prolapse of intraocular content; (2) deformation of the eyeball, and discontinuity of the eye ring with partially thickened eyeball wall, due to contusion-induced edema, laceration, or penetration (Fig. 3.1); (3) hematocele within the eyeball, revealed by increased density of the anterior or vitreous body (Fig. 3.2); (4) traumatic cataract, revealed by decreased density of the crystalline lens, or increased volume of the crystalline lens with deformation and rough edge (Fig. 3.3); (5) displacement of the crystalline lens (dislocation or prolapse), due to partial or complete rupture of the crystalline lens suspension ligament (Fig. 3.4); (6) foreign bodies or gas accumulation within the eyeball (Fig. 3.5); (7) combination with retinal detachment, revealed by slightly increased density of the posterior of the eyeball, with "V"-shaped margin pointed to the optic disc area (Fig. 3.6); and (8) sometimes combination with choroidal detachment, revealed by slightly increased density of shuttle or hemispherical shaped tissue (Fig. 3.7).
2. MRI scans: Deformation of the eyeball, thickened eye ring. MRI can show abnormal SI of the crystalline lens or mixed SI within the vitreous body alone with the increased time interval between the injury and scanning. Acute hemorrhage can represent as high SI.

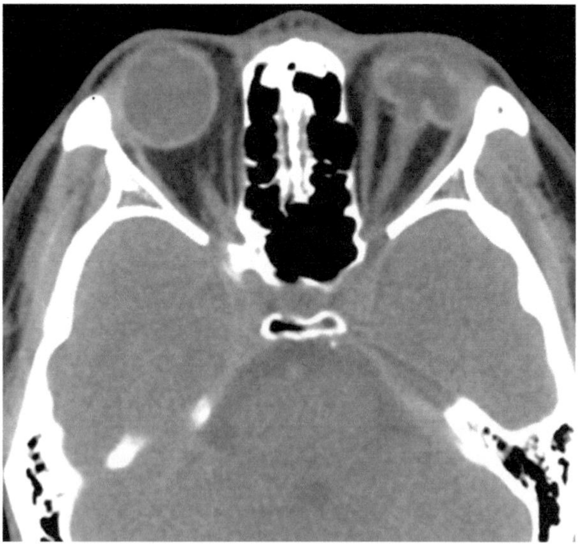

Fig. 3.1 Rupture of the left eyeball. Cross-sectional CT image in soft-tissue window showed the deformation of the left eyeball

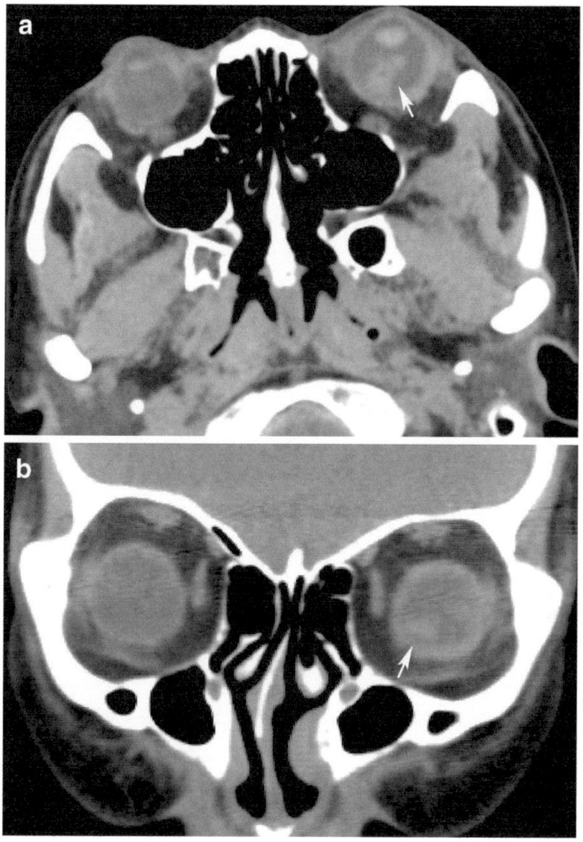

Fig. 3.2 Hemorrhage of the left vitreous body. (**a**) Cross-sectional CT image in soft-tissue window showed the irregular patchy high density within the left vitreous body (*arrow*), with normal shape and location of the crystalline lens. (**b**) Coronal CT image in soft-tissue window showed multiple patchy higher densities within the left vitreous body (*arrow*)

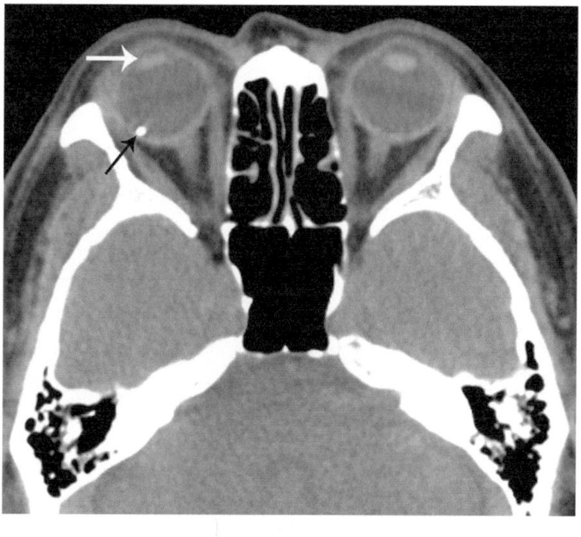

Fig. 3.3 Traumatic cataract of the right eye. Cross-sectional CT image in soft-tissue window showed decreased density of the right crystalline lens with deformation and blurred edge (*white arrow*), and a spherical foreign body with metal density in the posterior part of the eyeball (*black arrow*)

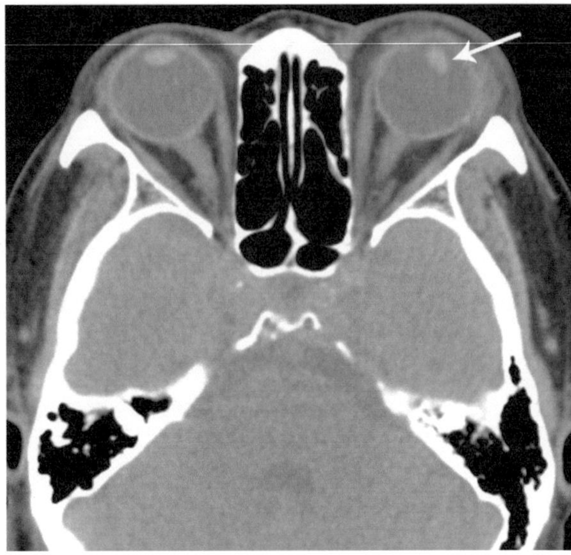

Fig. 3.4 Displacement of the left crystalline lens. Cross-sectional CT image in soft-tissue window showed abnormal location of the crystalline lens with relatively normal shape

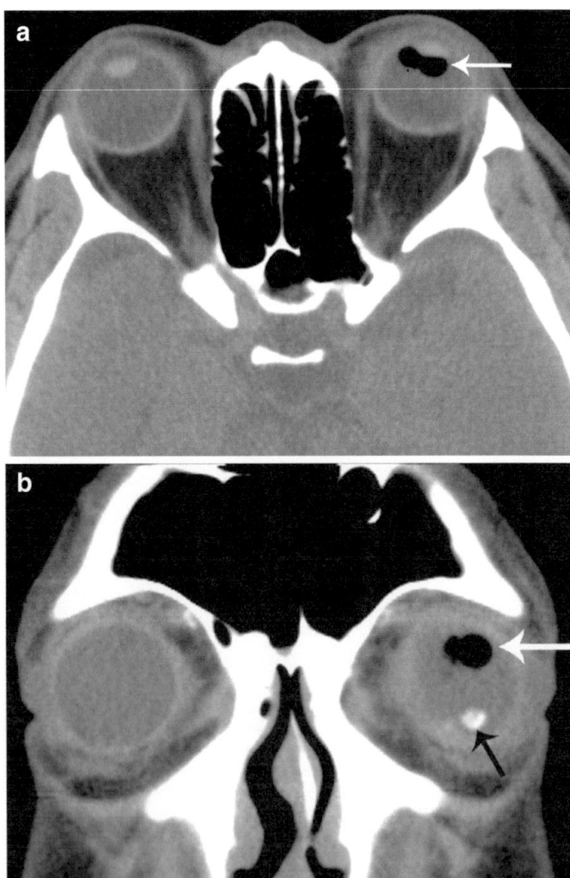

Fig. 3.5 Foreign bodies and gas accumulation within the eyeball. (**a**) Cross-sectional CT image in soft-tissue window showed gas density posterior to the crystalline lens of the left eye (*white arrow*). (**b**) Coronal CT image in soft-tissue window showed low-density gas (*white arrow*) and high-density foreign body (*black arrow*) within the left eye

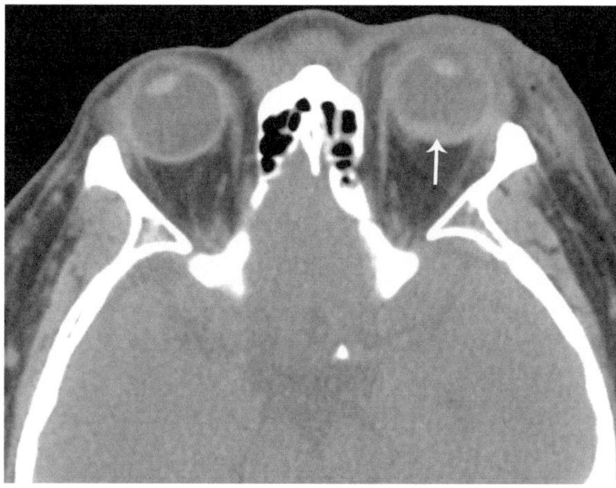

Fig. 3.6 Subretinal dropsy of the left eye. Cross-sectional CT image in soft-tissue window showed curve-shaped tissue with slightly higher density in the posterior part of the left eye (*white arrow*)

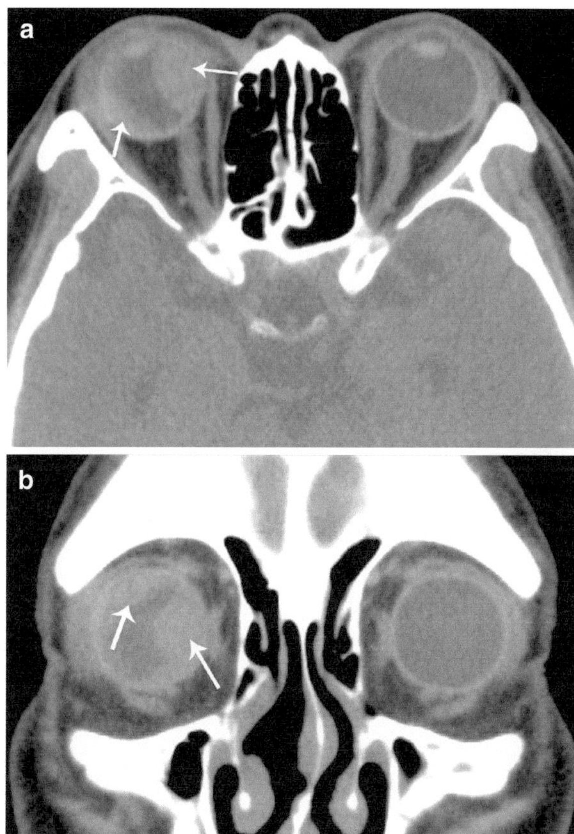

Fig. 3.7 Choroidal detachment and subchoroidal dropsy of the right eye. (**a**) Cross-sectional CT image in soft-tissue window showed clear margined shuttle and hemispherical shaped tissue with slightly higher density in the right eye (*white arrow*). (**b**) Coronal CT image in soft-tissue window showed shuttle and hemispherical shaped tissue with slightly higher density in the upper and nasal side of the right eye (*white arrow*)

3.1.4 Evaluation

Multi-slice spiral CT scan can show the severity of injury with high speed and accuracy. Bone window shows the fracture of orbital cavity and adjacent bones, providing more information to the clinician. MRI is characterized with high spatial resolution. However, it is not firstly recommended due to its longer scanning time and higher cost, except for those patients with suspected optic nerve or extraocular muscle injuries.

3.2 Soft-Tissue Injury

3.2.1 Pathological Features

1. Soft-tissue injury, mainly including injury of the optic nerve, extraocular muscles, lacrimal glands, hemorrhage and hematoma, eyelid swelling, and gas accumulation within the orbital cavity and eyelid.
2. Optic nerve injury, divided into two kinds: (1) primary injury, including break, contusion, compression of optic nerve sheath, and adjacent cavity by hemorrhage, and (2) secondary injury, including optic nerve edema, compression of the vessel, or circular obstacle.
3. Extraocular muscle injuries, including break, block, contusion, scar contraction, and adhesion.
4. Lacrimal gland injury, including edema, hemorrhage, and prolapse.
5. Hemorrhage within the orbital cavity can distribute separately in the soft tissue or present as hematoma. Subperiosteum hematoma is defined as hematoma between the orbital periosteum and bone.

3.2.2 Order of the Imaging Examination

1. CT scan: CT scan is the first choice due to its convenience, fast speed, and high-density resolution.
2. MRI scans: Its soft tissue resolution is superior to CT scan. It can clearly reveal the injury of the optic nerve, extraocular muscles, and hematoma within the orbital cavity, better than CT scan. If the optic nerve injury is suspected, the MRI scan should be performed as soon as possible for the sake of treatment. Metal foreign bodies are contraindications.

3.2.3 Radiologic Features

1. Optic nerve injury: CT scan cannot show the optic nerve injury clearly. The injured optic nerve can only present as thickening, blurred edge or discontinuity (Fig. 3.8). Hemorrhage of the optic nerve sheath and adjacent cavity represents as increased density (Fig. 3.9). Coronal view can show annular higher density around the optic nerve. Besides the altered shape of the optic nerve, the MRI scan can show increased SI on T2WI of it, indicating contusion and edema. The SI around the optic nerve can be varied in different time points of the hemorrhage. Typical manifestation is high SI on T1WI and T2WI around the optic nerve.

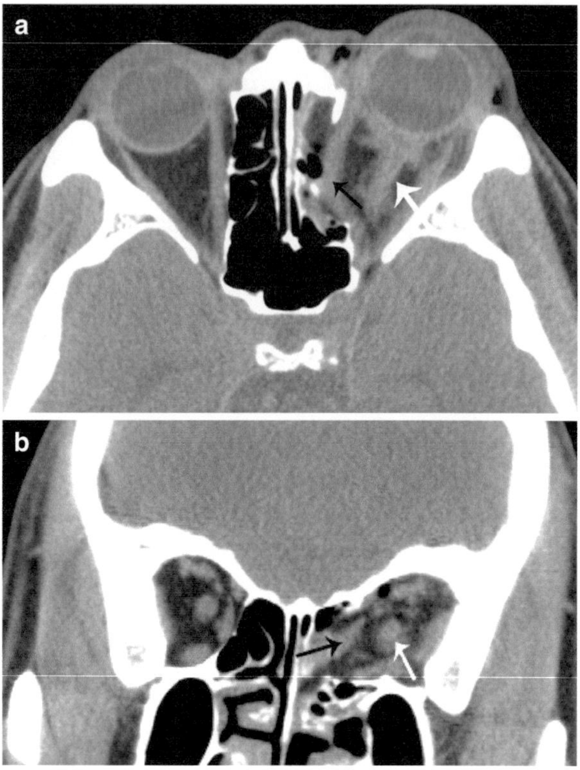

Fig. 3.8 Left optic nerve injury. (**a**) Cross-sectional CT image in soft-tissue window showed thickened left optic nerve with blurred margin (*white arrow*). It also showed fracture of the medial orbital wall displacing to the ethmoid sinus, combined with tortuous and displaced media rectus (*black arrow*). (**b**) Coronal CT image in soft-tissue window showed thickened left optic nerve (*white arrow*), with blurred fat space around. The abnormally shaped left media rectus partially displaced to the left ethmoid sinus (*black arrow*)

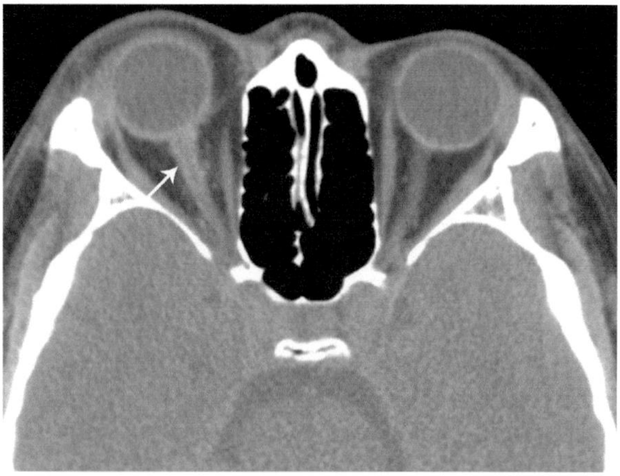

Fig. 3.9 Hemorrhage of the right optic nerve sheath. Cross-sectional CT image in soft-tissue window showed thickened right optic nerve with increased density of the margin (*arrow*)

2. Extraocular muscle injuries: CT and MRI scan can show the altered shape and location of the extraocular muscles, mainly including thickening, displacement, twist, or incarcerated to the fracture areas. (Fig. 3.8). When extraocular muscles are broken, the ruptured muscles are not always displayed on CT scan directly. Sometimes normal extraocular muscle is absent in the corresponding area, in this condition, the muscle break should be considered. (Fig. 3.10). MRI scan is superior to the CT scan due to the blurred fat space, spread edema, and hemorrhage. The lacerated and detached muscle tendon represented as mass can be showed clearly. The edema in the damage zone is present as (slightly) decreased SI on T1WI and high SI on T2WI. Hemorrhage within 2 weeks is present as high SI on both T1WI and T2WI, and its SI will be decreased as the time passes by. Scar with low SI and peripheral tissue adhesion will appear in the late stage of extraocular muscle injuries.
3. Lacrimal gland injury: CT images can show the increased volume of the lacrimal gland with blurred margin; increased density of the gland, which may due to hemorrhage; bone chips or foreign bodies in the gland; and the anterior and inferior displacement of the gland. MRI can show the edema (low SI on T1WI, high SI on T2WI) and hemorrhage (within 2 weeks, high SI on both T1WI and T2WI).
4. Hemorrhage in the orbital cavity: CT scan can show the blurred fat space retrospective to the eyeball, combined with patchy higher density (Fig. 3.11). Hematoma is present as oval or spindle-shaped, iso- or slightly high-density mass. Its MRI SI can be varied in different hemorrhage time points. Subperiosteum hematoma is present as spindle or flat mass along with the orbital wall, iso- or slightly high density, with clear border and without crossing the bone suture on the CT scan (Fig. 3.12). On the MRI, the SI variation of subperiosteum hematoma is same as that of hemorrhage: slightly low SI in the super acute and acute phase; slightly high SI in the subacute phase; and low SI on T1WI and high SI on T2WI in the chronic phase.

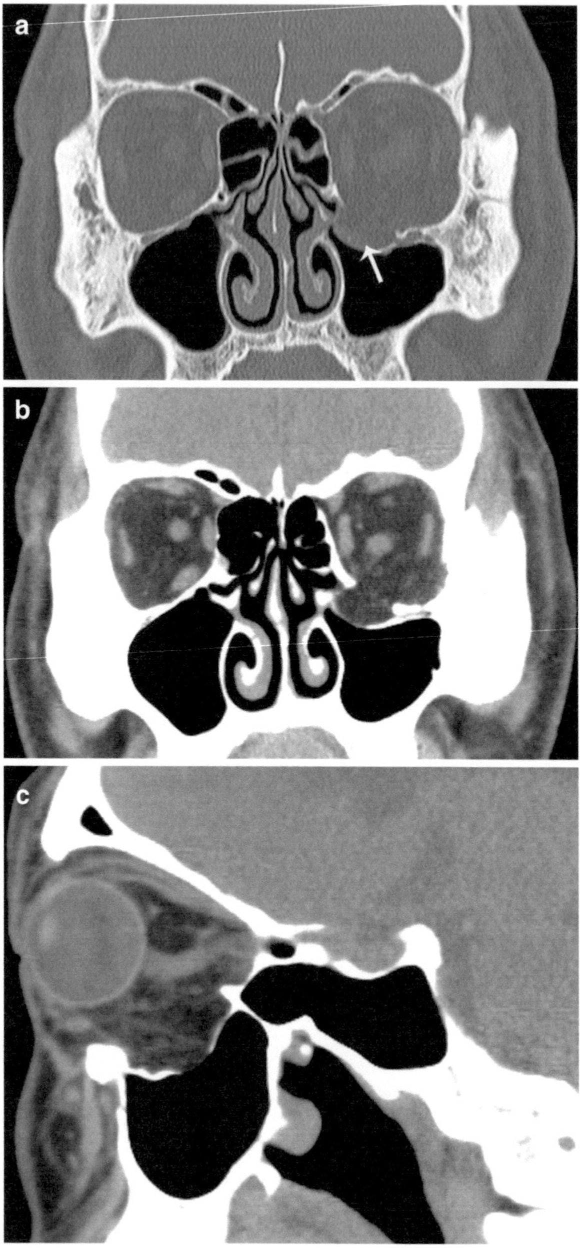

Fig. 3.10 The fracture of left inferior orbital wall combined with inferior rectus break (injured 4 years ago, *upper* strabismus of the eye). (**a**) Coronal CT image in bone window showed discontinuity of the left inferior orbital wall (white arrow). (**b**) Coronal CT image in soft-tissue window showed the fat within the left orbital cavity protruded in the maxillary sinus. The left inferior rectus was absent. (**c**) Oblique sagittal CT image in soft-tissue window showed the absence of the left inferior rectus

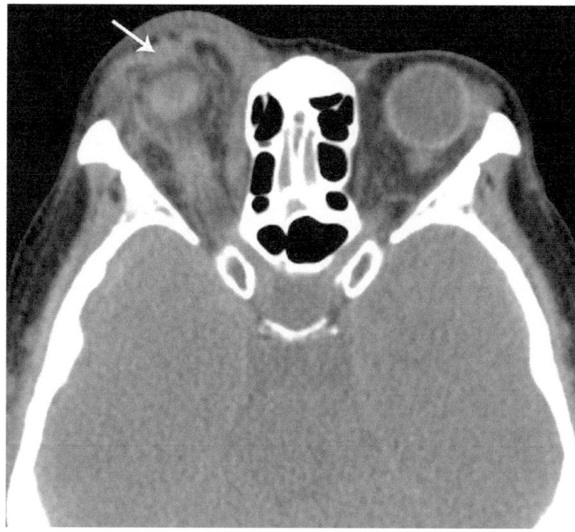

Fig. 3.11 Hemorrhage in the right orbital cavity. Cross-sectional CT image in soft-tissue window showed blurred fat space in the right orbital cavity, combined with patchy slightly high density (*white arrow*)

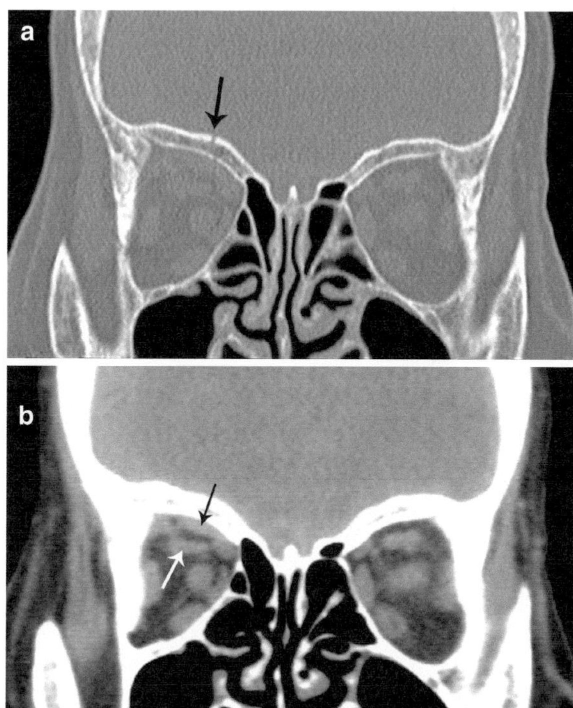

Fig. 3.12 Fracture of the right superior orbital wall combined with subperiosteum hematoma. (**a**) Coronal CT image in bone window showed discontinuity of the right superior orbital wall without significant dislocation (*black arrow*). (**b**) Coronal CT image in soft-tissue window showed a slightly high-density mass in spindle shape with clear margin, along with the superior orbital wall (*black arrow*). This is the subperiosteum hematoma. The superior group of the extraocular muscle is compressed and displaced inferiorly (*white arrow*)

3.2.4 Evaluation

Multi-slice spiral CT scan can show most of the orbital soft-tissue injury. The bone window can demonstrate whether there is any fracture of the orbital and adjacent bones, providing essential diagnostic information in the early stage. MRI is characterized with high spatial resolution. It is sensitive to soft-tissue contusion, edema, and early-stage optic nerve injury. For the break of extraocular muscle, which is hard to be determined on CT scan, MRI can show its priority than CT in providing information to clinicians.

3.3 Orbital Wall Fracture

Severe collision injuries usually lead to orbital wall fractures. The injuries can lead to swelling and bruising of the eyelid, protruded eyeball, limitation of movement of the eyeball, followed by enophthalmus, diplopia, movement disorder, impaired vision, and even blindness. Enophthalmus and diplopia are typical manifestations of blowout fracture (Niu et al., 2013).

3.3.1 Order of the Imaging Examination

1. CT scan: CT image is of high-density resolution. Multiplane reconstruction of the spiral CT is considered as the best method, because it can reveal the soft tissue and orbital bone clearly.
2. MRI scans: MRI can show the soft tissue better than CT. But it is not sensitive to fracture.

3.3.2 Radiologic Features

1. CT scan: The medial orbital wall fracture is the most common manifestation (Fig. 3.13), followed by the inferior orbital wall (Fig. 3.14). The adjacent intra-orbital soft tissue can protrude into ethmoid sinus or maxillary sinus. The affected extraocular muscle can be swelling, thickening, tortuous, with blurred margin and increased density. The gas from adjacent nasal sinus can move into the orbital cavity through the fracture, leading to intra-orbital gas accumulation (Fig. 3.15). The normal fat space between the extraocular muscle and medial orbital wall can be narrowed or disappeared (Fig. 3.13c). The extraocular muscle can block into the collapse place of the fracture (Fig. 3.8). There are slightly high density and hematoma in the adjacent ethmoid and maxillary sinus. The rupture of the small vein in the orbital cavity can lead to hematoma or hemorrhage (Fig. 3.10). The fracture of orbital apex can affect the optic nerve canal and injure the optic nerve.

   It is quite important to differentiate newly and dated fracture, because the diagnosis of fracture is usually related with disputes and forensic identification. CT manifestation of dated orbital fracture includes depression of the orbital wall with smooth and continued margin (Fig. 3.10); extraocular muscle can be thickened, but with clear border; fat space adjacent to the fracture does not show blurring significantly; endophthalmos can be seen, without acute manifestations such as gas accumulation in the orbital cavity and swelling eyelid, etc. (Fig. 3.16).

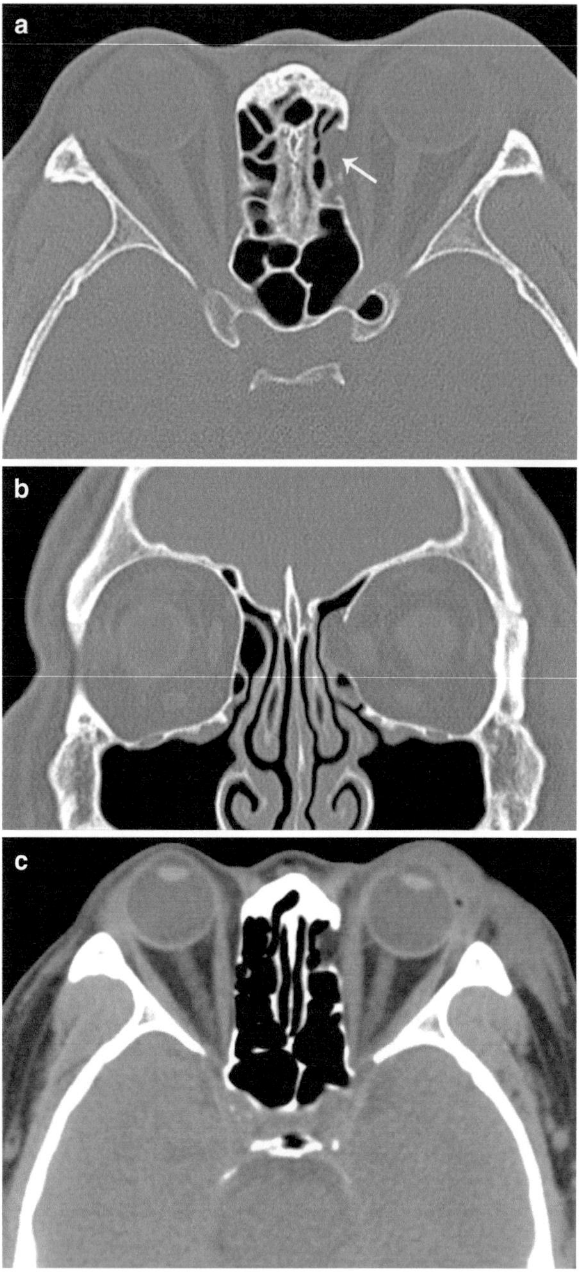

Fig. 3.13 Fracture of the left medial orbital wall. (**a**) Cross-sectional CT image in bone window showed the discontinuity of the left medial orbital wall (*white arrow*), part of the intra-orbital soft tissue protruded into ethmoid sinus. (**b**) Coronal CT image in bone window showed the discontinuity of the left medial orbital wall. (**c**) Cross-sectional CT image in soft-tissue window showed thickened medial rectus with blurred margin. The fat space between the medial rectus and medial orbital wall is blurred and narrowed. The left eyelid and temporal soft tissue are swelling.

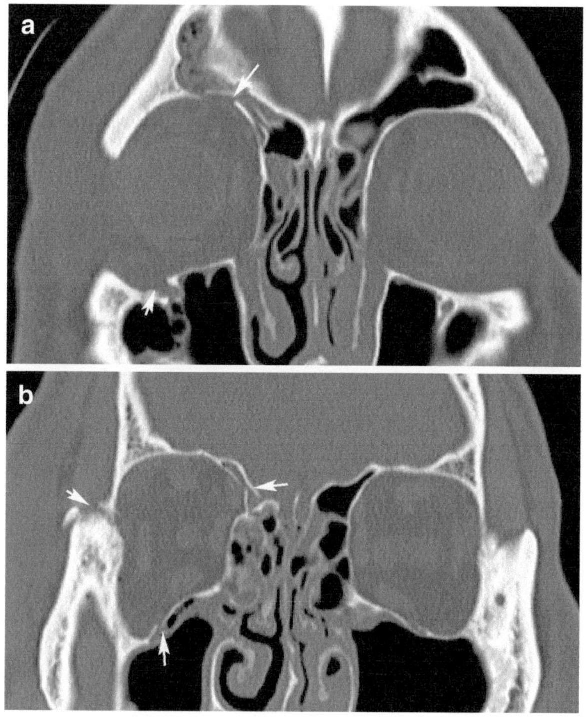

Fig. 3.14 Fracture of each side of the right orbital wall. (**a**) Coronal CT image in bone window showed fracture of the right superior (*long arrow*) and inferior (*short arrow*) orbital wall. The inferior orbital cannel is affected. (**b**) Coronal CT image in bone window showed fracture of right lateral, inferior, and medial orbital wall. The inferior orbital canal and medial-superior corner were affected. Hematocele within the ethmoid sinus was also present

2. MRI scans: Abnormal shape of the orbital wall with discontinuity of the SI. MRI can also present other abnormalities such as encephalomeningocele, subperiosteum hematoma, and hematoma in the orbital cavity.

3.3.3 Evaluation

Before the invention of CT, doctors applied plain film in Caldwell-Water position to diagnose orbital fracture. But the diagnosis was often missed or late due to the overlaid orbital structures and the low resolution of the plain film. Now this method is rarely used.

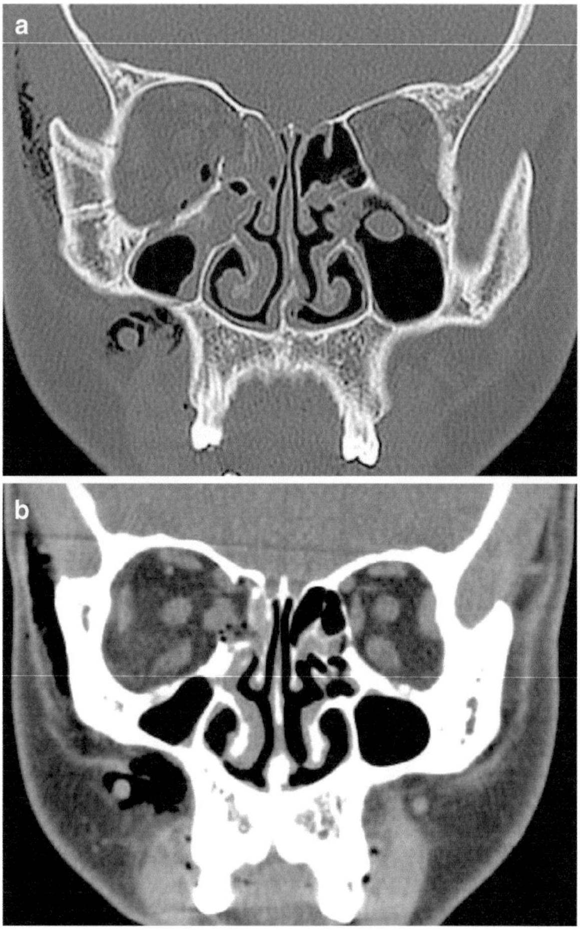

Fig. 3.15 Orbital cavity injuries induced fractures and secondary alternations. (**a**) Coronal CT image in bone window showed discontinuity of the right medial orbital wall, and the medial-superior and medial-inferior corner were all affected. Gas accumulated in the orbital cavity, temporal fossa, and infratemporal fossa. (**b**) Coronal CT image in soft-tissue window showed part of the soft tissue in the orbital cavity protruded into the ethmoid sinus. The medial rectus and superior oblique muscle were thickened and partially blocked. Slightly high density could be seen in the right ethmoid sinus.

Cross-sectional CT scan could reveal the fracture of medial and lateral wall and tissue within the orbital cavity accurately. But for the superior and inferior orbital wall, their linear fracture cannot be shown well due to their parallel position to the scanning position. Coronal CT scan is vertical to orbital wall, so that it can show the details of each side. So both cross-sectional and coronal CT scans are recommended when the orbital wall fracture is suspected. Spiral CT can acquire the cross-sectional images, and then reconstruct the coronal images. Thus we can early diagnose the fractures and reduce the rate of missed diagnosis.

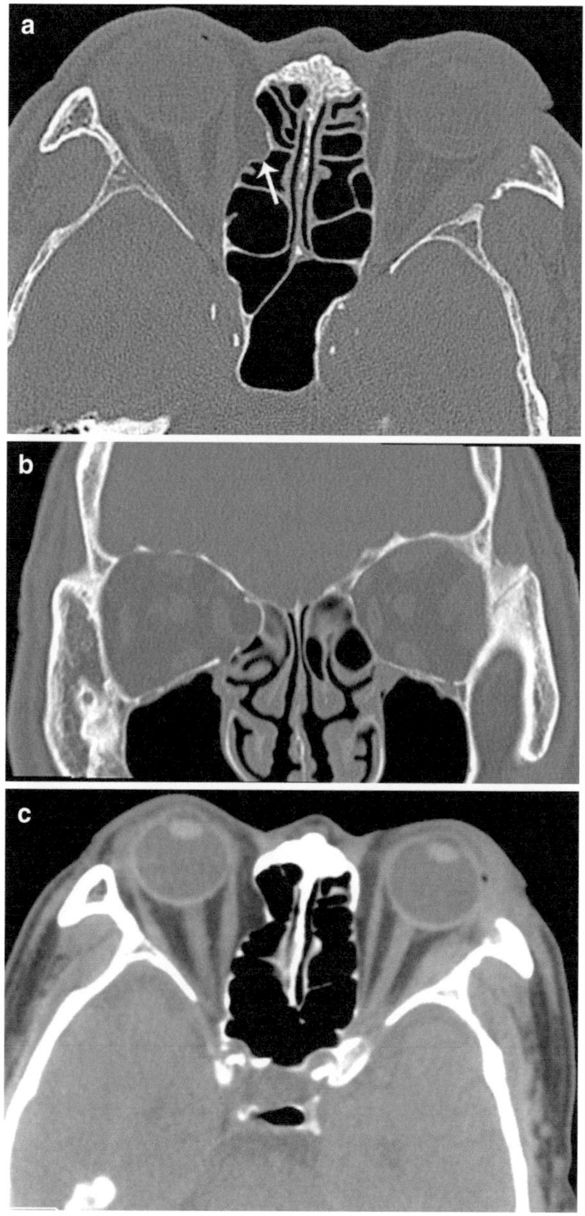

Fig. 3.16 Dated fracture of the right medial orbital wall. (**a**) Cross-sectional CT image in bone window showed fracture of the right medial orbital wall. The wall was protruded into the ethmoid sinus. Its margin is clear (*arrow*). (**b**) Coronal CT image in bone window showed similar results. (**c**) Cross-sectional CT image in soft-tissue window showed slightly thickened medial rectus with clear border. The fat space between the muscle and medial orbital wall is clear

3.4 Fracture of the Optic Nerve Cannel

3.4.1 Order of the Imaging Examination

1. CT scan: Multi-slice spiral CT scan is the first choice used to diagnose the fractures of the optic nerve cannel.
2. MRI scans: It is useless when diagnosing the fractures. But it is needed when optic nerve injury is suspected.

3.4.2 Radiologic Feature

1. CT scan: Multi-slice spiral CT scan with cross-sectional, coronal, and sagittal plan reconstruction or conventional HRCT cross-sectional and coronal scan can increase the diagnostic rate of the fractures of the optic nerve cannel. Cross-sectional CT scan of the optic nerve cannel can demonstrate discontinuity of the medial and lateral wall (Fig. 3.17). Coronal scan can demonstrate well continuity of each side of the wall (medial, lateral, superior, inferior) (Fig. 3.18). Oblique sagittal scan can demonstrate the superior and inferior wall. The fracture can be diagnosed on the cross-sectional and coronal scan, or based on combination of scans in three directions. We also need to observe whether there are bone chips within or adjacent to the optic nerve cannel, or fractures of the skull base (Hart and Zimmer 2008).

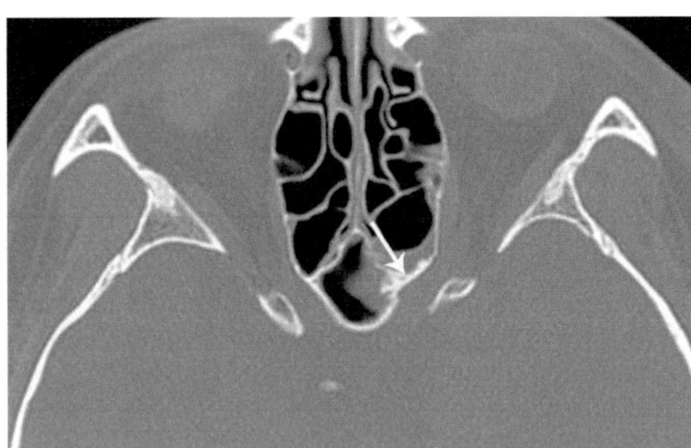

Fig. 3.17 Fracture of medial wall of the left optic nerve canal. Cross-sectional CT image in bone window showed discontinuity of the medial wall of the left optic nerve cannel (*white arrow*).

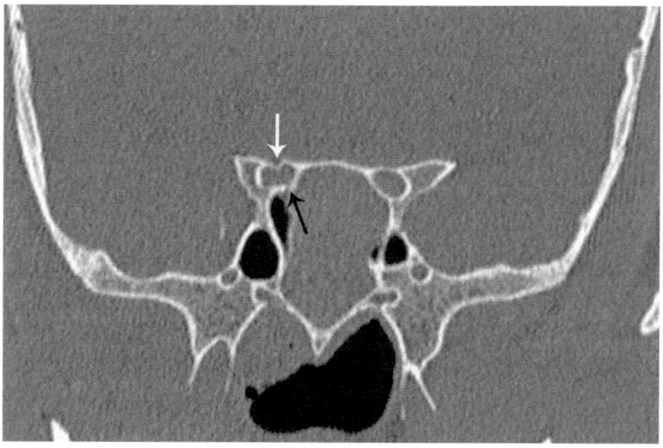

Fig. 3.18 Fracture of superior and inferior wall of the right optic nerve cannel. Coronal CT image in bone window showed discontinuity of the superior (*white arrow*) and inferior (*black arrow*) of the right optic nerve cannel

3.4.3 Evaluation

HRCT scan is the first choice used to diagnose the fractures of the optic nerve cannel. The combination of cross-sectional, coronal scan (and oblique sagittal reconstruction) can increase the detection rate of fracture of each side of the optic nerve cannel. If hematoma within the optic nerve cannel or optic nerve injury is suspected, MRI scan is needed.

3.5 Foreign Body Within the Orbital Cavity

3.5.1 Pathological Features

1. The main pathological feature of the foreign body within the eyeball is the penetrating wound of the eye. The direct injury of the eye can induce secondary infection.
2. The degree of secondary injury and pathological changes is related with the characteristic and size of the foreign body. The foreign bodies usually include iron, bronze, stone, bits of wood or glass, etc. Metal foreign body can lead to atrophy of the eyeball due to its chemical injury. Nonmetal foreign body often induces infective inflammation.
3. Simple foreign body, located within the orbital cavity but beyond the eyeball, induced secondary alternations that are relatively simple, which are similar to those within the eyeball (Fezza and Wesley 1999).

3.5.2 Order of the Imaging Examination

1. X-ray: It is the conventional method to diagnose the foreign body within the orbital cavity which is easily applied in basic hospitals.
2. Ultrasound: Ultrasound can clearly demonstrate the foreign body within the eyeball and eyeball wall, but it is not sensitive to the foreign body within the orbital cavity.
3. CT scan: CT scan is of high resolution. The diagnostic capacity of multiplane reconstruction CT images is significantly superior to the X-ray.
4. MRI scans: The nonmetal foreign body and its complications can be shown on MRI images, better than that on CT. Metal foreign body is the contraindication.

3.5.3 Radiologic Features

1. X-ray: Foreign body often presents as irregularly shaped with halation around. It is considered within the eyeball if it is located in the radius of 10 mm of the orbit center on the posteroanterior view of the plain film, and in the distance of 20 mm to the front margin of the orbital cavity. Otherwise it is considered beyond the eyeball. The clinicians usually use the Балтцн method to locate the foreign body (Fig. 3.19).
2. Ultrasound: Hypo-echoic light can be seen in the vitreum. Metal or stone is present as strong-echoic light spot or facula. Foreign body such as plastic and glass is present as hyper-echoic light spot or facula.

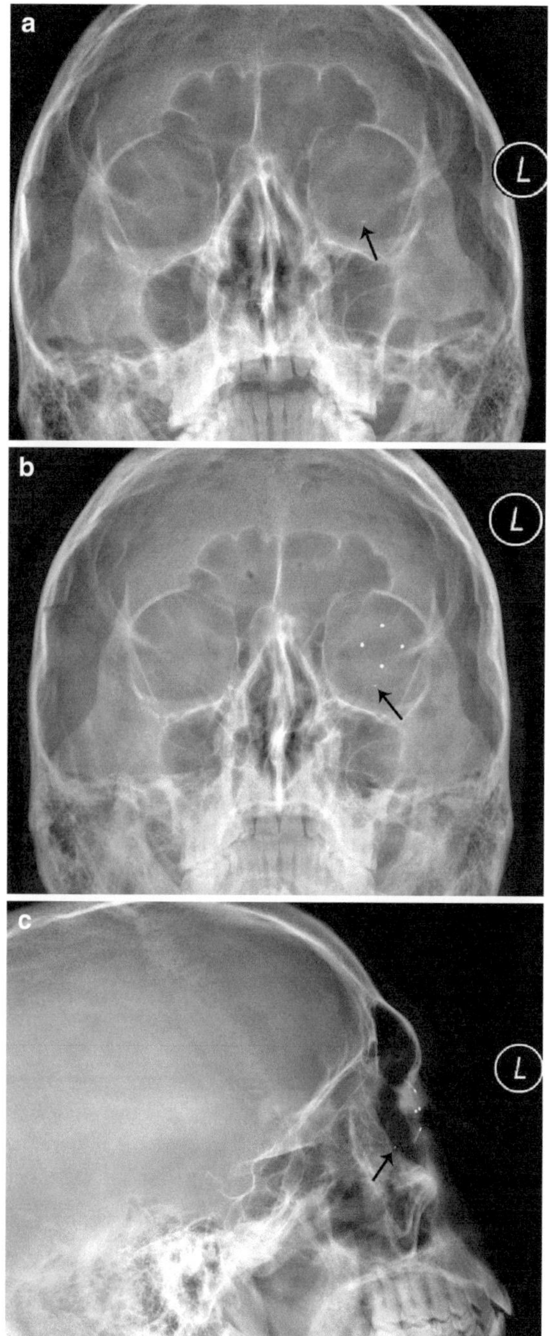

Fig. 3.19 Foreign body in the left orbital cavity. (**a**) The posteroanterior view of the plain film showed patchy high density in the left orbital cavity (*black arrow*). (**b**) The posteroanterior view using the Балтцн method showed a distance of 14 mm from the foreign body to the center of the eyeball. (**c**) The lateral view using the Балтцн method showed a distance of 11 mm from the foreign body to the margin of cornea

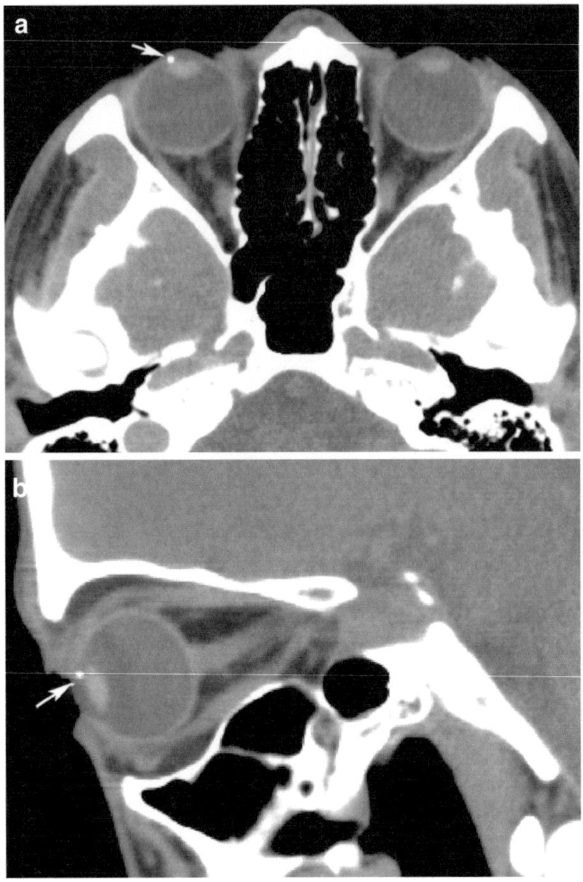

Fig. 3.20 Foreign body within the right eyeball. (**a**) Cross-sectional CT scan without contrast enhancement showed a dot-shaped high-density foreign body in the temporal side of anterior chamber of the right eye (*white arrow*). (**b**) Reconstructed sagittal CT image showed a dot-shaped high density in the superior part of the anterior chamber

3. CT scan: CT can find foreign body in the anterior chamber, crystal, vitreum, eyeball wall, or other places in the orbital cavity. Different texture may present as different density. There are significant artifacts around large metal foreign body. Indirect signs include alternations of direct injury of the soft tissue in the orbital cavity, such as thickened eye ring induced by penetration, swelling, density decreasing, deformation and displacement of the crystal, and abnormal shape and density of the intra-orbital fat tissue, optic nerve, and extraocular muscles (Figs. 3.20, 3.21, 3.22, 3.23, and 3.24a).
4. MRI scans: Metal foreign body is contraindication. Nonmetal foreign body represents as abnormal SI within or beyond the eyeball. It is well shown on T2WI. Indirect signs include vitreous hemorrhage, endophthalmitis, and atrophy

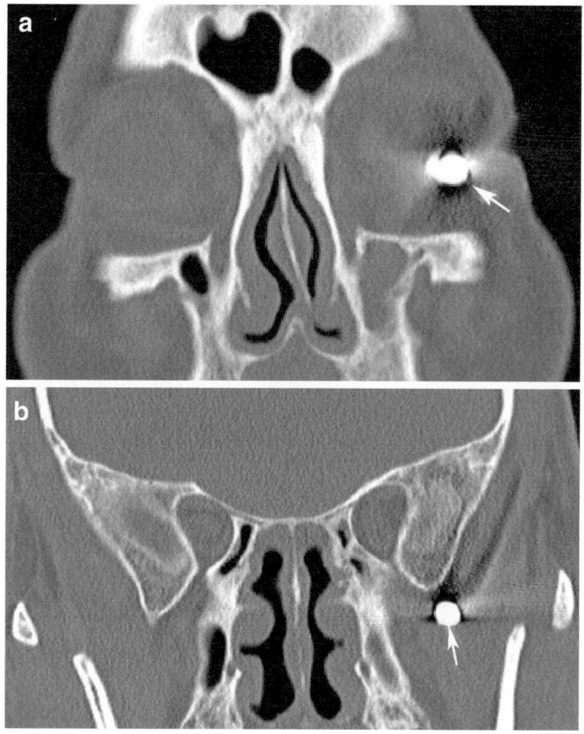

Fig. 3.21 Foreign body in the left orbital cavity. (**a**) Coronal CT image in bone window showed a round-shaped high density in the left orbital wall (a part of concrete iron falls down and inserts into the orbital cavity). (**b**) Coronal CT image in bone window showed the foreign body in the left orbital cavity inserted into the left infratemporal fossa (*white arrow*)

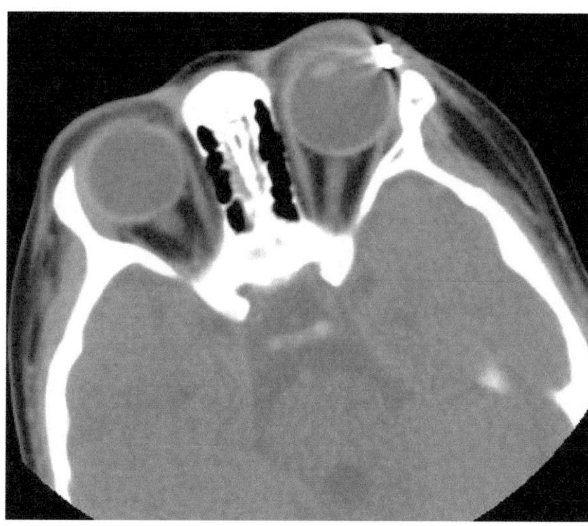

Fig. 3.22 Foreign body in the left orbital cavity. Cross-sectional CT image in soft-tissue window showed a nodular shaped high density anterior to the left eyeball in the temporal side

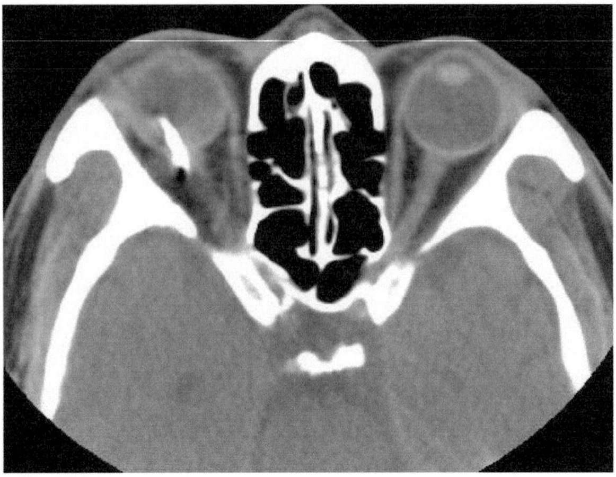

Fig. 3.23 Foreign body in the right eyeball. Cross-sectional CT image in soft-tissue window showed a strip-shaped high density in the posterior part of the right eyeball, partially protruded out of it. Fat space posterior to the right eyeball was unclear. Right crystalline lens was not clear

of eyeball. If combined with inflammation, there is striking contrast after contrast administration between the significantly enhanced inflammatory lesion and unenhanced foreign body (Fig. 3.24b–d).

3.5.4 Evaluation

Foreign body in the orbital cavity is one of the most common kinds of injury of the eye. It will lead to serious consequences if not treated in time. Some metal foreign bodies can remain in the eye and induce severe chemical reactions with adjacent tissue. It is very important to determine the location and characterization of the foreign body when selecting the operation method. The prognosis evaluation is directly associated with the characterization, location, and adjacent injuries of the foreign body. X-ray is cheap and easy to be used. But it is not sensitive to those small-sized radiopaque foreign bodies or radiolucent foreign bodies. Ultrasound can clearly demonstrate the foreign body within the eyeball and eyeball wall, but it is not sensitive to the foreign body within the orbital cavity. CT is the first choice due to its high resolution and multiplane reconstruction ability. The nonmetal foreign body and its complications can be shown on MRI images, better than on CT. But MRI scan is a supplementary choice due to its high cost and long scanning time.

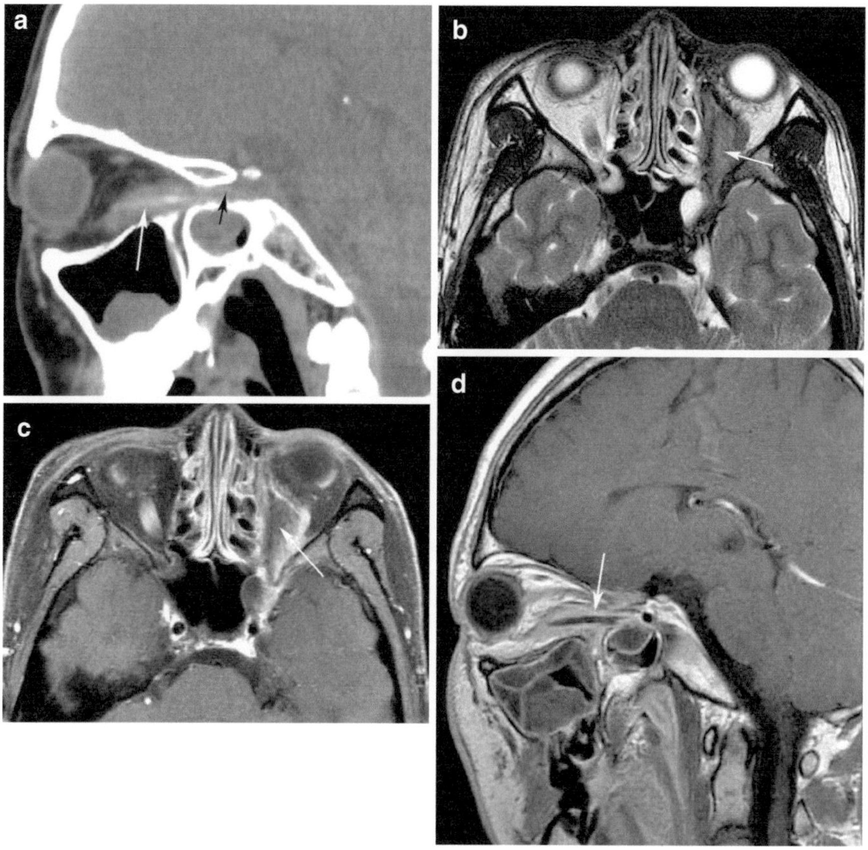

Fig. 3.24 Foreign body combined with inflammation. (**a**) Sagittal CT image without contrast enhancement showed an anteroposterior-positioned soft tissue with mixed density and blurred margin. A strip-shaped slightly high density was seen in the center of the lesion (*white arrow*), extended to the superior orbital fissure (*black arrow*). (**b**) Cross-sectional MR image showed an irregular shaped, mixed iso- to slightly high SI tissue on T2WI, extended to the cavernous sinus through the superior orbital fissure. (**c**) After contrast agent administration, the tissue was shown with inhomogeneous enhancement on the cross-sectional fat-suppressed image. The left superior orbital fissure and cavernous sinus were widened and enhanced. (**d**) Oblique sagittal MRI scan showed moderate inhomogeneous enhancement after contrast. The foreign body in the center remained unenhanced (*white arrow*)

References

Fezza J, Wesley R. The importance of CT scans in planning the removal of orbital-frontal lobeforeign bodies. Ophthalmic Plast Reconstr Surg. 1999;15(5):366–8.

Hart CK, Zimmer LA. Computed tomography anatomy of the Optic Canal. Otolaryngol Head Neck Surg. 2008;139(2):139–74.

Niu Y, Li B, Li C, et al. Analysis of eye injury situation and causes of orbital blow-out fracture. International Eye Science. 2013;13(2):374–6.

Chapter 4
Inflammatory Diseases

Han Lv, Zhenchang Wang, and Zhengyu Zhang

4.1 Cellulitis and Abscess

Orbital cellulitis is a kind of acute inflammatory disease of the soft tissue in the orbital cavity induced by bacterial infection, often secondary to sinusitis or trauma, commonly seen in children. The clinical manifestations are including: redness and swelling of the eyelid, conjunctival congestion and edema, eye movement disorder, may be combined with vision loss. If the inflammation was not controlled in time, it could lead to superior ophthalmic vein thrombophlebitis, intraorbital abscess, and thrombophlebitis, meningitis, subdural abscess if there's intracranial involvement.

4.1.1 Pathological Features

1. A large amount of neutrophil infiltration in the loose connective tissue.
2. The superior orbital phlebitis can lead to intraorbital abscess, and cavernous sinus thrombophlebitis, meningitis, subdural abscess if there's intracranial involvement (Mouriaux et al. 2012).

H. Lv • Z. Wang (✉)
Department of Radiology, Beijing Friendship Hospital, Capital Medical University, Beijing, China
e-mail: cjr.wzhch@vip.163.com

Z. Zhang
Department of Radiology, Beijing Unicare ENT Hospital, Beijing, China

Z. Wang et al. (eds.), *Diagnostic Imaging of Ophthalmology*,
https://doi.org/10.1007/978-94-024-1060-0_4

4.1.2 Order of the Imaging Examination

1. Ultrasound: Ultrasound is the first choice. It is an easy used and fast examination.
2. CT scan: CT image can demonstrate abnormal alternations of the soft tissue and adjacent bone.
3. MRI scans: MRI is of high soft tissue resolution. It can clearly show the extent of disease.

4.1.3 Radiologic Features

1. Ultrasound: The fat pad posterior to the eyeball is enlarged with inhomogeneous echoes and sparse spots on ultrasound imaging. Crack is present between the eyeball wall and the fat pad. There are characteristics of tenonitis if the tenon capsule is involved.

2. CT scan: Eyelid is swelling. In the early stage of nasal source infection, the lesion is restricted in the extra space of the extraocular muscle cone space. The medial rectus is thickened with blurred margin. Along with the progression of the disease, it will present as exophthalmos, the fat space of orbital septum, intra- and extraocular muscle cone space will be disappeared and filled by soft tissue. The extraocular muscles are thickened and suppressed in vague density. The eyeball wall, optic nerve and lacrimal gland can be involved. The hyperplasia and hardening of the orbital wall are due to long time, repeated inflammation stimulation. CT can demonstrate the bone of orbital wall better than MRI. The thickened and enhanced meningeal is present if the intracranial space is involved. The wall of abscess is significantly enhanced (Figs. 4.1a, 4.2, and 4.3a).

3. MRI scans: The inflammation in the early stage is only confined in the extraocular muscle cone space. There is soft tissue SI (iso-SI on T1WI and high SI on T2WI) with blurred boundary in medial part of the orbital cavity adjacent to the nasal sinus. The sinusitis is usually seen. Along with the progression of the disease, the margin of normal anatomic structures disappeared, combined with swelling of the eyelid, thickening of extraocular muscles with blurred margin, widespread mixed SI in the intra- and extraocular muscle cone space, which is low SI on T1WI, mixed high SI on T2WI, widespread inhomogeneous enhanced on fat-suppressed T1WI, and multiple abscess cavities in different sizes (Fig. 4.1b–d, Fig. 4.3b–d). Subperiosteal abscess is characterized as

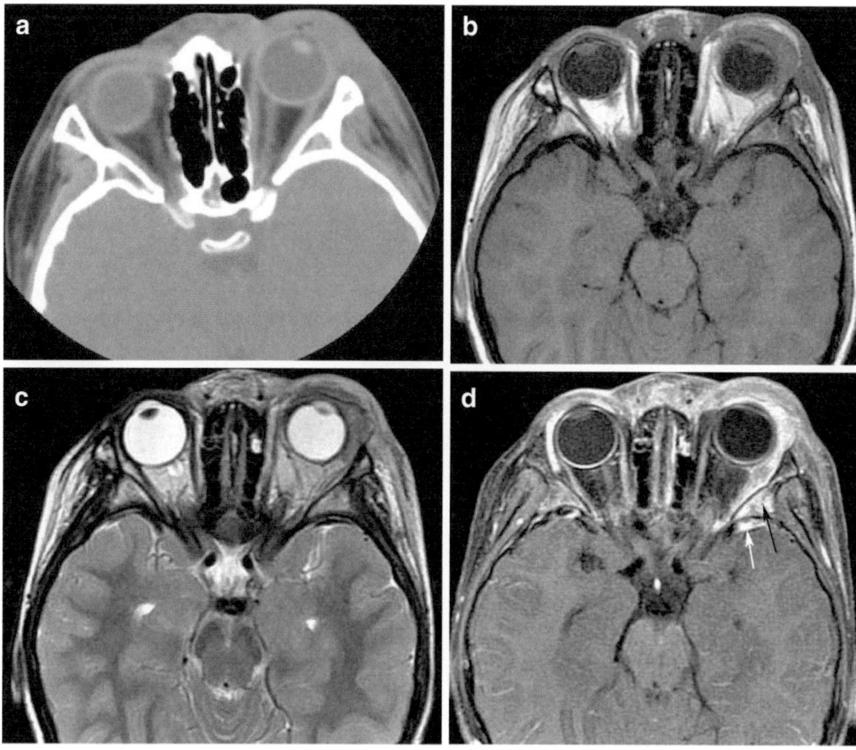

Fig. 4.1 Cellulitis in the left orbital cavity. (**a**) Cross-sectional CT image in soft tissue window showed widely swelling and thickening of left eyelid, soft tissue on the left temporal and back of nose regions. (**b**) Cross-sectional T1WI without enhancement administration showed the blurred margined lesion with inhomogeneous slightly lower SI. (**c**) Cross-sectional T2WI showed mixed inhomogeneous hyper-intensity. (**d**) After contrast enhanced, the cross-sectional MR image showed inhomogeneous enhanced lesion, which was extended to superior orbital fissure posteriorly. The boundary between the lesion and lacrimal gland was not clear. The temporal pole meningeal was thickened and enhanced (*white arrow*). There was patchy of enhancement in the greater wing of sphenoid bone (*black arrow*)

wide substrate abnormal SI (iso- or slightly low SI on T1WI, high SI on T2WI) under the orbital wall with clear or blurred margin. The edge of the lesion is homogeneously enhanced, and the center remains unenhanced. When there is venous thrombus, the SI of the vein will be increased and the flow void signal disappeared. The orbital cellulitis can be intracranial spread and combined with severe complications such as cavernous sinus thrombophlebitis, meningitis, subdural abscess, and sepsis. The meninges and the abscess wall are significantly thickened and enhanced (Kapur et al. 2009).

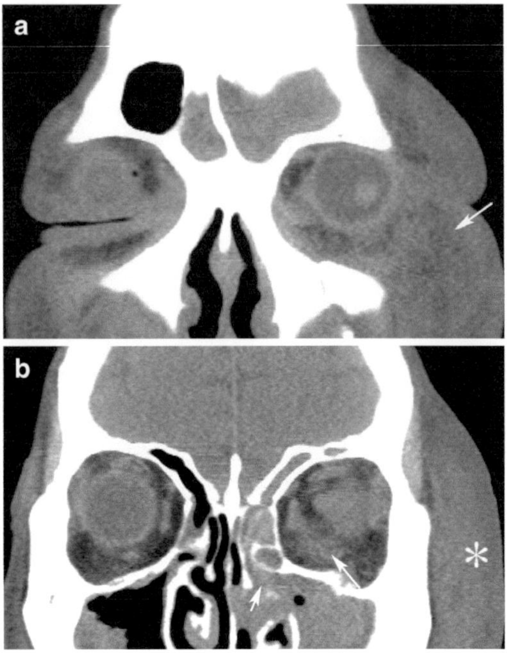

Fig. 4.2 Cellulitis in the left orbital cavity. (**a**) Coronal CT image in soft tissue window showed widely swelling and thickening of the left temporal and facial soft tissue (secondary inflammation due to inappropriate management after trauma) (*white arrow*). (**b**) Coronal CT image in soft tissue window showed swelling of the left zygomaticofacial soft tissue (asterisk) and widely distributed cable strip shadow in the intra- and extraocular muscle cone space with blurred margin (*long arrow*). There was soft tissue in the left ethmoid sinus and maxillary sinus (*short arrow*)

4.1.4 Evaluation

The diagnostic value of traditional X-ray is limited. Ultrasound is a noninvasive examination. It is fast and easy to be used, which can indicate the pathological stage according to the altered echo. But it cannot observe abnormalities deep in the orbital cavity, nor can reveal alternations adjacent to the lesion. CT and MRI scans can comprehensive and objective display the range of lesion and adjacent structures and combined osteomyelitis, sinusitis, foreign body, etc. They are important methods used for the clinical diagnosis and therapeutic evaluation of orbital cellulitis. The diagnosis and differential diagnosis of cellulitis are based on combination of clinical history, clinical manifestation, and radiologic manifestations.

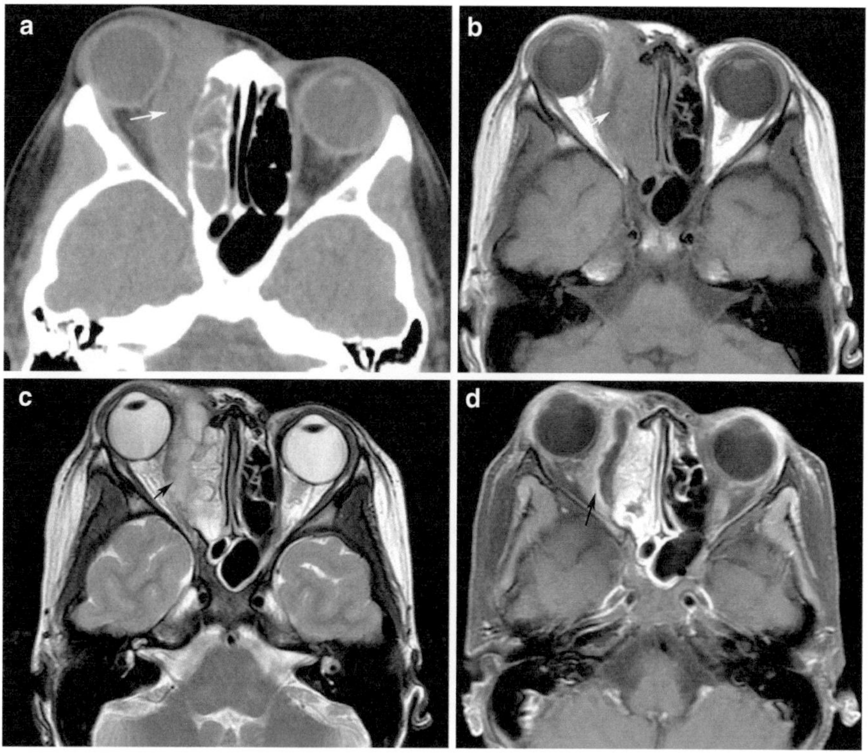

Fig. 4.3 Subperiosteal abscess secondary to nasal source cellulitis in the right orbital cavity. (**a**) Cross-sectional CT image in soft tissue window showed strip shaped soft tissue in the nasal side of right orbital cavity, which is not separate from the medial rectus. The adjacent ethmoid sinus was filled with soft tissue density. (**b**) Cross-sectional T1WI without enhancement showed inhomogeneous iso-intensity lesion with strip shaped hypo-intensity in the center. The lesion in the orbital cavity and the ethmoid sinus were not separated clearly. The fat in the extraocular muscle cone space disappeared. (**c**) Cross-sectional T2WI showed mixed hyper-intensity in the right orbital cavity and ethmoid sinus. The medial rectus was thickened with increased SI, which was not separated from the lesion. (**d**) Cross-sectional contrast enhanced T1WI with fat saturation showed significant inhomogeneous enhanced lesion in the orbital cavity, with strip shaped unenhanced part in the center. The lesion in the right ethmoid was significantly enhanced

4.2 Idiopathic Orbital Inflammation

4.2.1 Pathological Features

1. Lymphocytic infiltration type: Scattered distributed or infiltrated with large amount of lymphocytes, plasma cells, and (or) eosinophilic cells.
2. Constrictive type: Hyperplasia of large amount of fibrous connective tissue placed in rope or clumps shape. Parts of the lesion are hyaline changed or degenerated. Only small amount of lymphocytes and (or) plasma cells infiltrated.
3. Mixed type: Represent as mixed fibrous connective tissue with infiltrated and hyperplastic chronic inflammation cells. Collagen fiber wraps around the lesion. Parts of the collagen fiber are hyaline changed or degenerated (Mouriaux et al. 2014).

4.2.2 Order of the Imaging Examination

1. Ultrasound. Ultrasound can reveal the structure, characterization of the lesion and its relationship with adjacent soft tissue.
2. CT scan. CT can show the shape, size, location of the lesion and spatial positioning it. It can also show the secondary changes around the lesion. CT scan is recommended.
3. MRI scans. MR images can show the lesion clearly. It can indicate the structure of the lesion according to its different SI.

4.2.3 Radiologic Features

1. Ultrasound: The results are complicated. The echoic features are varied according to the growth pattern and involved structures. If the lesion grows like a mass, it can be a mass shaped lesion with clear margin, low echo-level inside, and blurred posterior margin, which can arise from both the intra- and the extraocular muscle cone space. For the diffused inflammation, the lesions are widespread in the orbital cavity and involve multiple structures. The lesions show inhomogeneous echoes on ultrasound imaging. Structures in the orbital cavity cannot be identified clearly. Lesion arises from the lacrimal gland, presents with enlarged lacrimal gland with decreased echo-level inside and clear posterior boundary. The extraocular muscle involvement can represent as thickened one or multiple extraocular muscles, including the swelling of the tendon attachment points.

2. CT scan: Multi-slice spiral CT scan can clearly show the scope and involved structure of the inflammatory pseudotumor. The lesion is of multiple manifestations without a specific feature. It is mainly in inhomogeneous soft tissue density and inhomogeneous enhanced. If the lesion grows like a mass, it can be a mass shaped lesion in soft tissue density with clear margin, located in any part of the orbital cavity. The adjacent extraocular muscle is suppressed and displaced with blurred margin. The eye ring will be thickened, combined with irregular shape of the eyeball and relatively homogeneous enhancement if the eyeball wall and tendon attachment points are involved. For the diffused inflammation, there is diffused soft tissue posterior to the eyeball, which is hardly differentiated with other structures. The low density of intraorbital fat will be disappeared, combined with thickened optic nerve with blurred margin, and increased density and enlargement of both the eyelid and orbital part of lacrimal gland if involved. If the extraocular muscles are involved, there will be diffused enlargement of multiple extraocular muscles with blurred margin. The tendon attachment points are thickened as well.
3. MRI scans: The MRI scans can not only clearly show the shape and scope of the lesion, but also can determine its pathological type according to its SI. If the mass is iso-intensity on both T1WI and T2WI, it may be the lymphocytic infiltration type. If the mass is slightly low-intensity on both T1WI and T2WI, it may be due to hyperplasia of fibrous connective tissue. Diffused inflammatory lesion is present as irregular mass with blurred margin in the orbital cavity, poorly differentiated with adjacent structures. When the lacrimal gland and extraocular muscles are involved, they will not only show enlargement, their SI can also be altered similar to the lesion. Both the muscle belly and tendon are thickened. The lesions are inhomogeneous moderate enhanced (Fig. 4.4, Fig. 4.5).

4.2.4 Evaluation

B-type ultrasound can observe the lesion in different aspects. It can determine a solid or cystic lesion by pressing the detector to observe whether there is nerviness. Thus it can be differentiated with hemangioma or dermoid cyst. But the ultrasound cannot clearly show and locate the lesion deeper more than 4 cm to the orbital margin, nor the bone destruction.

The CT and MRI features of the inflammatory pseudotumor are varied and lack specific features. It should be diagnosed with close combination of the clinical history.

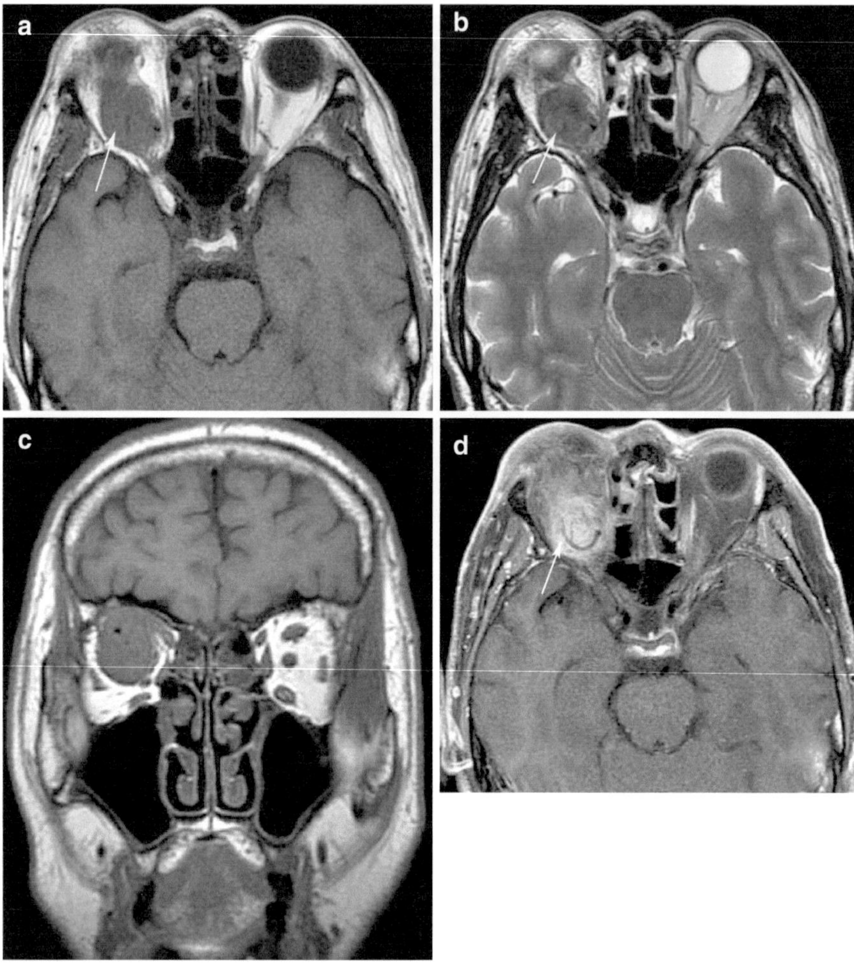

Fig. 4.4 Inflammatory pseudotumor in the right orbital cavity. (**a**) Cross-sectional T1WI without contrast enhancement showed an irregular shaped mass in iso-intensity with clear margin in the right orbital cavity (*white arrow*). The eyelid is swelling and thickened. (**b**) Cross-sectional T2WI showed the lesion is of low-intensity with inhomogeneous SI (white arrow). (**c**) Coronal T1WI without contrast enhancement showed both the intra- and extraocular muscle cone space were involved. There was no crack between the lesion and superior extraocular muscle group and superior oblique muscle. The optic nerve was compressed and moved downward. (**d**) Cross-sectional MRI after contrast administration showed inhomogeneous moderate enhancement of the lesion with flow void vessel inside

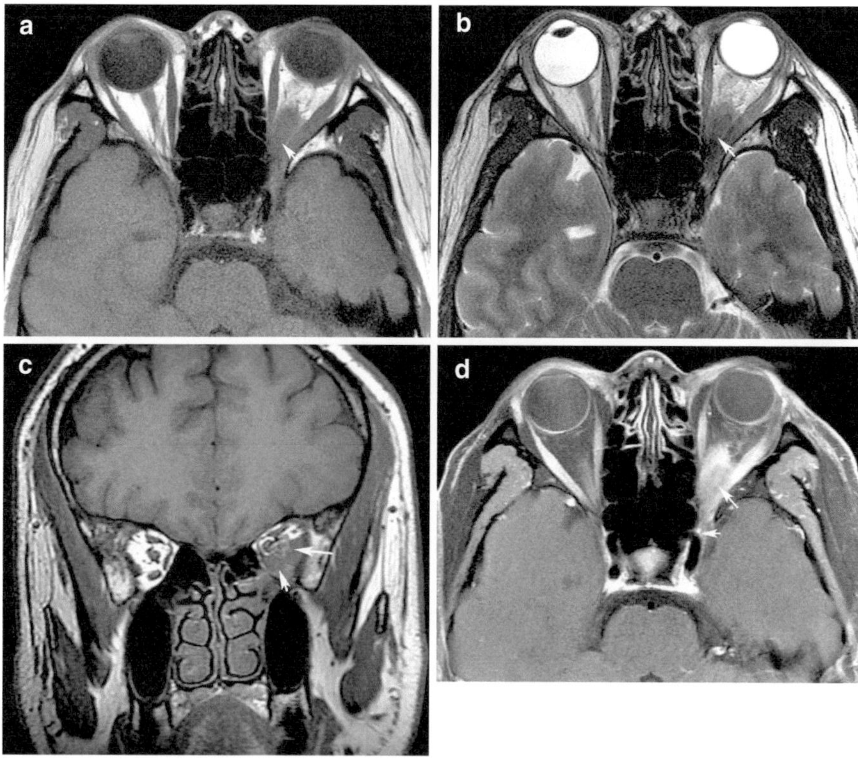

Fig. 4.5 Inflammatory pseudotumor in the left orbital cavity. (**a**) Cross-sectional T1WI without contrast enhancement showed an iso-intense soft tissue in the left orbital apex (*white arrow*), which was poorly differentiated with other structures of the orbital apex. (**b**) Cross-sectional T2WI showed slightly low SI of the lesion (*white arrow*). The cavernous sinus was involved through the enlarged superior orbital fissure. (**c**) Coronal T1WI without contrast enhancement showed the involvement of inferior rectus (*short arrow*) and lateral rectus (*long arrow*). The muscle bellies were thickened significantly and poorly differentiated with the lesion. The margin of optic nerve was blurred. (**d**) Cross-sectional MRI with fat saturation after contrast administration showed moderate enhanced lesion in the left orbital apex (*long arrow*). The cavernous sinus was involved through the enlarged superior orbital fissure (*short arrow*). (The clinical manifestation was painful ophthalmoplegia with significant restriction of ocular upward and inward rotation. The lesion was reduced in volume in the reexamination after 3 months of hormone treatment)

4.3 Graves Disease

Graves disease is a thyroid related ocular disease associated with multiple factors when the thyroid functions are normal. It may be related with gene, autoimmunity, and other factors. The ocular disease is also a tissue specific autoimmunity disease. The main clinical manifestations are including: painless proptosis and ophthalmoplegia, often bilaterally involved. The onset of disease is occult. Half of the patients had no symptom or had only light symptoms. They always visit the doctors after the disease found by others. The course of disease is short. Graves disease is more commonly seen in female (Bartalena 2013).

4.3.1 Pathological Features

1. Present as edema of extraocular muscles and chronic inflammation cells (including lymphocytes, plasma cells) infiltration in the early stage of disease. Mainly affect the muscle belly. Few can affect the tendon.
2. Present as fibrosis of extraocular muscles combined with partially fatty degeneration in the late stage of disease.
3. Increased fat tissue posterior to the eyeball within the orbital cavity, combined with diffused inflammatory changes.

4.3.2 Order of the Imaging Examination

1. MRI scans: It can demonstrate not only the altered shape of extraocular muscles, but also the abnormal SI to infer the stage of disease indirectly. MRI scans are the first choice. The widened superior ophthalmic vein, subarachnoid space broadening, and increased optic disc area are all indications of compression of orbital apex by the thickened extraocular muscles.
2. CT scan: Multi-slice spiral CT scan with multi-plane reconstruction can clearly show the thickened extraocular muscles in spindle shape.

4.3.3 Radiologic Features

1. CT scan: Exophthalmos and thickened extraocular muscles in spindle shape (Fig. 4.6). There is no significant alternation of the tendon and its stopping point, nor does the thickened eye ring. The compression of ophthalmic vein will lead to congestion and widening. It can combine with edema of conjunctiva and eyelid or enlargement of the lacrimal glands.

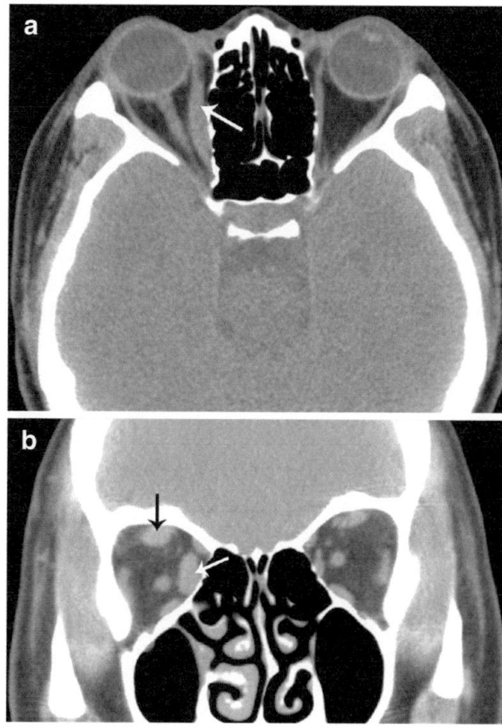

Fig. 4.6 Right sided Graves disease. (**a**) Cross-sectional CT image in soft tissue window showed thickened right medial rectus (*white arrow*) in spindle shape. (**b**) Coronal CT image in soft tissue window showed the thickened superior extraocular muscle group (*black arrow*) and medial rectus (*white arrow*)

2. MRI scans: Usually present as thickening of multiple extraocular muscles, or thickening of one muscle. The rank of incidence is inferior, medial, superior, and lateral rectus. The thickening part mainly occurred in the muscle belly (Fig. 4.7, Fig. 4.8). It can be either high or low SI due to the edema, fibrosis, and fatty degeneration of the extraocular muscles. They are obviously seen on T2WI. It can also present secondary changes such as thickened optic nerve and widened superior ophthalmic vein.

4.3.4 Evaluation

The CT scan is commonly used to diagnose Graves disease in clinical. The orbital CT can evaluate the size of extraocular muscles and locate the eyeball, which is helpful for the diagnosis of Graves disease. But CT scan cannot demonstrate minimal lesions, nor can differentiate the edema and fibrosis of extraocular muscles due to its lower resolution than MRI scans. The MRI scans can accurately locate the lesion and infer the stage of disease. Thus, the MRI scans are the first choice when Graves disease is suspected.

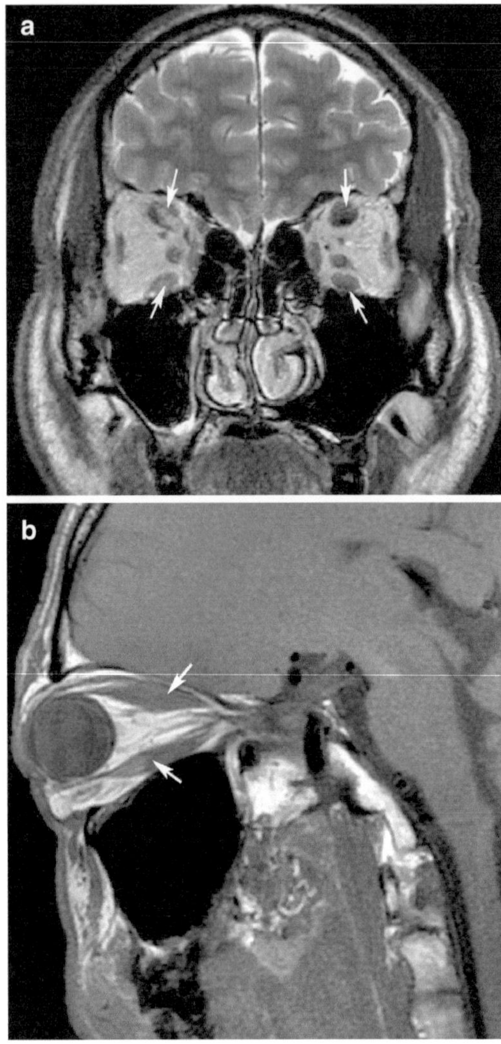

Fig. 4.7 Bilaterally Graves disease. (**a**) Coronal T2WI showed thickened bilateral superior extraocular muscle groups and inferior rectus, mainly affect the superior rectus. There was strip like high SI in the superior rectus. (**b**) Sagittal T1WI without contrast showed thickened superior and inferior rectus. The muscle bellies were mainly affected. The tendons were spared

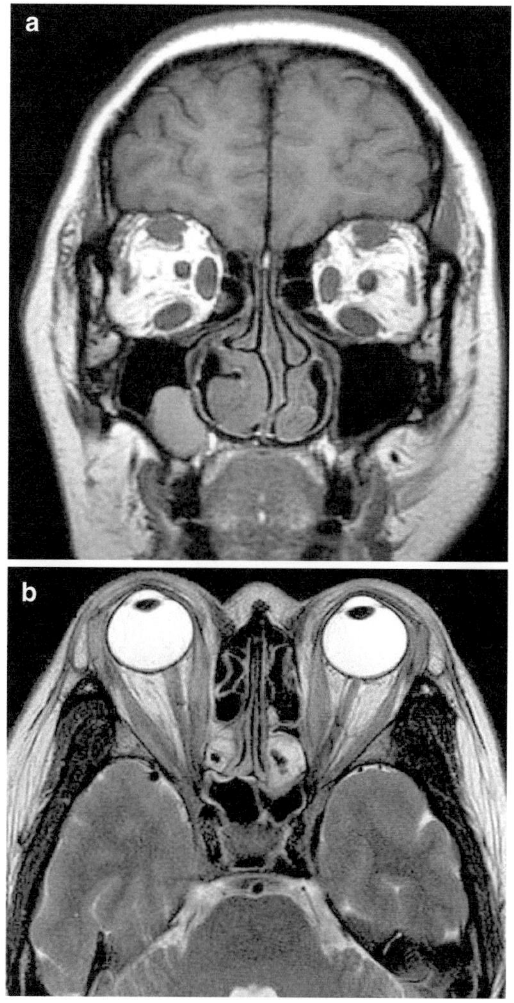

Fig. 4.8 Bilaterally Graves disease. (**a**) Coronal T1WI without contrast showed thickened bilateral medial, inferior rectus and superior extraocular muscle groups. (**b**) Cross-sectional T2WI showed thickened bilateral medial rectus and right lateral rectus. The muscle bellies were mainly affected

References

Bartalena L. Diagnosis and management of Graves disease: a global overview. Nat Rev Endocrinol Nat Rev Endocrinol. 2013;9(12):724–34.

Kapur R, Sepahdari AR, Mafee MF, et al. MR imaging of orbital inflammatory syndrome, orbital cellulitis, and orbital lymphoid lesions: the role of diffusion-weighted imaging. AJNR Am J Neuroradiol. 2009;30(1):64–70.

Mouriaux F, Rysanek B, Babin E, et al. Orbital cellulitis. J Franais Dophtalmol. 2012;35(1):52–7.

Mouriaux F, Pichonnet SC, Robert PY, et al. Orbital inflammation. J Franais Dophtalmol. 2014;37(10):818–24.

Chapter 5
Lymphoproliferative Lesions of the Orbit

Xinyan Wang, Junfang Xian, and Zhengyu Zhang

Orbit lymphoproliferative lesions originate from the lymphocytes of the orbit, eyelids, and conjunctiva, characterized by diffuse hyperplasia of small lymphocytes (Haradome et al. 2014).

5.1 Pathological Features

1. *Inflammatory pseudotumor.* Mature lymphocytes, plasmacytes, neutrophilic granulocytes, acidophilic cell endotheliocytes and varying amounts of endotheliocytes and fiber composition are visible.
2. *Reactive lymphocyte hyperplasia.* Diffuse mature small lymphocytes or mature follicle, and small amounts of plasmacytes and endotheliocytes can also be seen.
3. *Untypical lymphocyte hyperplasia.* Diffuse infiltration of lymphocytes which are mainly mature small lymphocytes is accompanied by different amounts of large to medium-sized lymphocytes. Nuclear multilobation may be present.
4. *Malignant lymphoma.* Widespread distribution of immature lymphocytes is visible, and nuclear multilobation may be present (Talaulikar et al. 2010).

X. Wang • J. Xian (✉)
Department of Radiology, Beijing Tongren Hospital, Capital Medical University, Beijing, China
e-mail: cjr.xianjunfang@vip.163.com

Z. Zhang
Department of Radiology, Beijing Unicare ENT Hospital, Beijing, China

Z. Wang et al. (eds.), *Diagnostic Imaging of Ophthalmology*,
https://doi.org/10.1007/978-94-024-1060-0_5

5.2 Imaging Protocols

1. Ultrasound

   Ultrasound can show the internal structure and blood of the lesion and relationship between the lesion and adjacent structures.
2. CT

   CT can display the lesion morphology, size, and location clearly, and spatial localization can be done. Furthermore, secondary changes of adjacent structures can be shown by CT.
3. MRI

   MRI shows the lesion more clearly, and tissue components of the lesion can be indicated according to different signal intensities on MR imaging.

5.3 Imaging Findings

Imaging findings of inflammatory pseudotumor is described in Sect. 4.2 of Chap. 4.

1. Ultrasound

   Ultrasound shows the lesion as a round or irregular, ill-defined and hypoechoic or echoless solid mass with moderate sound transmission. The mass can be compressed and posterior border is clearly visible.
2. CT findings

   Most lesions are irregular and well defined with unsmooth margin located in the outer upper quadrant of the orbit. The density of the inflammatory pseudotumor is usually homogenous with rare calcification and necrosis. When the tumor locates adjacent to the eyeball, it encases the eyeball demonstrating "casting mould" (Fig. 5.1a, b). The eyelids and adjacent subcutaneous soft tissue are commonly involved with blurred fat interspace, but the internal structure is often spared.
3. MRI findings

   Most lesions locate in the lacrimal gland and palpebral region, or may involve the orbit structures diffusely. Most inflammatory pseudotumors which are ill defined and irregular show homogenous isointense on T1WI and homogenous iso- or minimal hyperintense on T2WI. The lesions are prone to growth anteriorly and involve the extra-orbit structures or involve the extra-orbit structures along orbit holes. Reactive lymphocyte hyperplasia shows isointense on T1WI and T2WI and mild-moderate enhancement. Its enhancement is lower than that of inflammatory pseudotumor in which mainly are hyperplasia lymphocytes. Untypical lymphocyte hyperplasia (Fig. 5.2) is difficult to differentiate from lymphoma (Figs. 5.1 and 5.3) by growth pattern and MR findings.

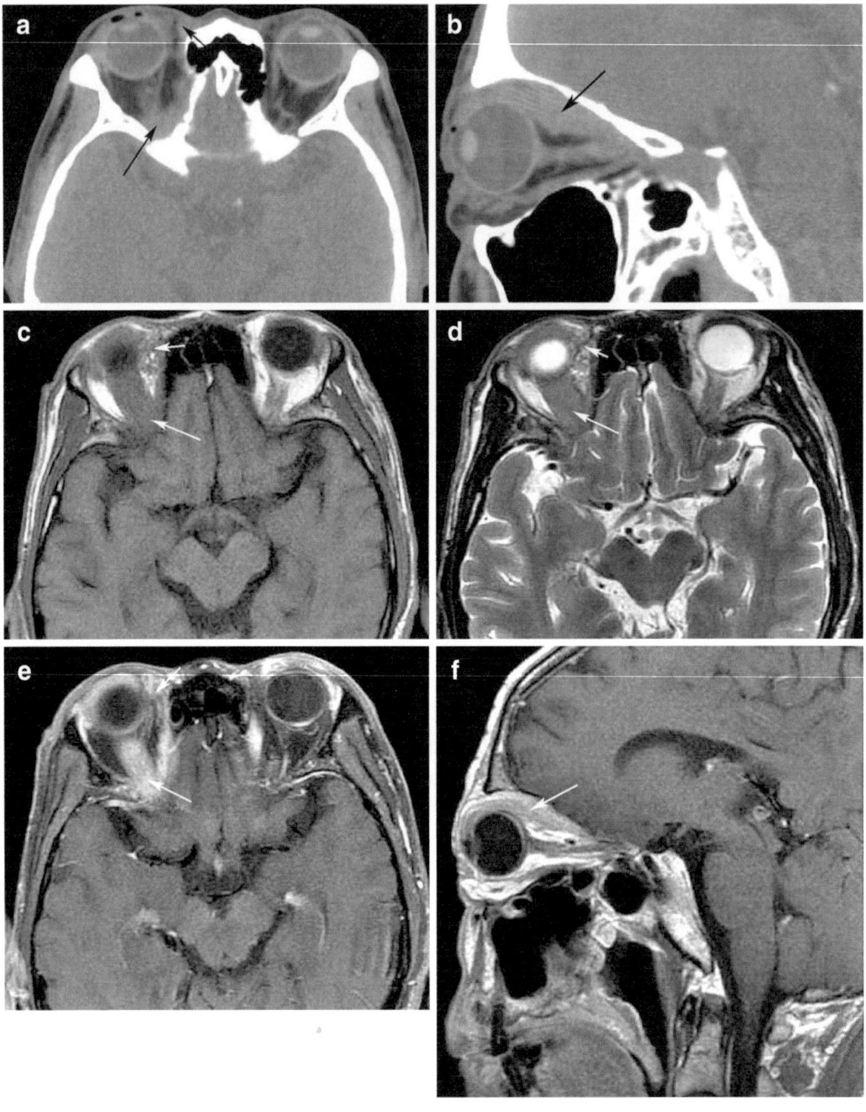

Fig. 5.1 Lymphoma in the right orbit. (**a**) Axial unenhanced CT with a soft tissue algorithm shows an irregular soft tissue mass in the upper quadrant of the right orbit (*long black arrow*) adjacent to orbit wall with intraconal and extraconal space involved. The lesion extend anteriorly with medial angle and nasal dorsum involved (*short black arrow*). (**b**) Sagittal unenhanced CT with a soft tissue algorithm shows the lesion extending into the orbital apex region in an anterior-posterior pattern adjacent orbit wall with levator palpabrae muscle and superior rectus involved and eyeball encased partially. (**c**) Axial T1-weighted MR image shows the thickening levator palpabrae muscle and superior rectus with isointense signal. The lesion encased the eyeball partially and involved the medical angle (short white arrow) with adjacent skin thickened. (**d**) Axial T2-weighted MR image shows the lesion isointense and ill-defined. (**e**) Axial contrast-enhanced MR image with fat saturation shows the lesion with moderate homogenous enhancement (*long white arrow*). The eyeball wall is thickened and enhances significantly. The lesion in the medical angle shows heterogeneous enhancement. (**f**) Sagittal contrast-enhanced MR image shows the mass with moderate homogenous enhancement

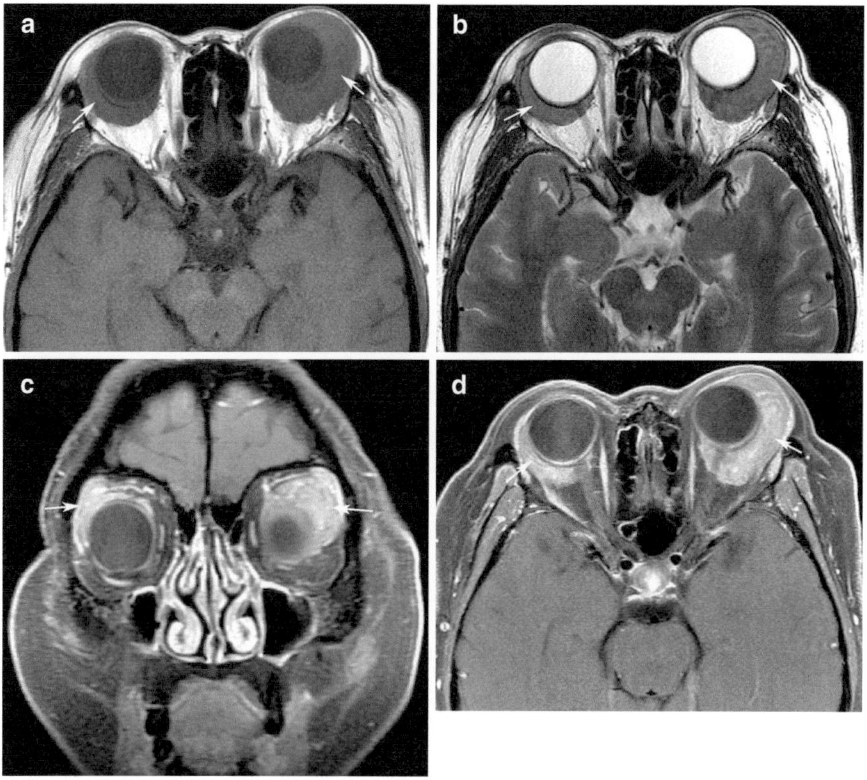

Fig. 5.2 Lymphoma in bilateral orbits. (**a**) Axial T1-weighted MR image shows the bilateral eyeballs are encased by bracket-shaped masses with slightly low signal intensity. The inner margin of the mass is undistinguishable from the eyeball wall, and the outer margin is smooth. (**b**) Axial T2-weighted MR image shows the lesions surrounding the eyeball with slightly low signal intensity. (**c**) Coronal contrast-enhanced MR image with fat saturation shows the tumor with heterogeneous moderate enhancement with punctiform and linar more significant enhancement in the middle part. (**d**) Axial contrast-enhanced MR image with fat saturation shows heterogeneous moderate tumor enhancement with punctiform and linar significant enhancement in the middle part. Bilateral lacrimal glands are compressed thinly and undistinguishable from the lesion

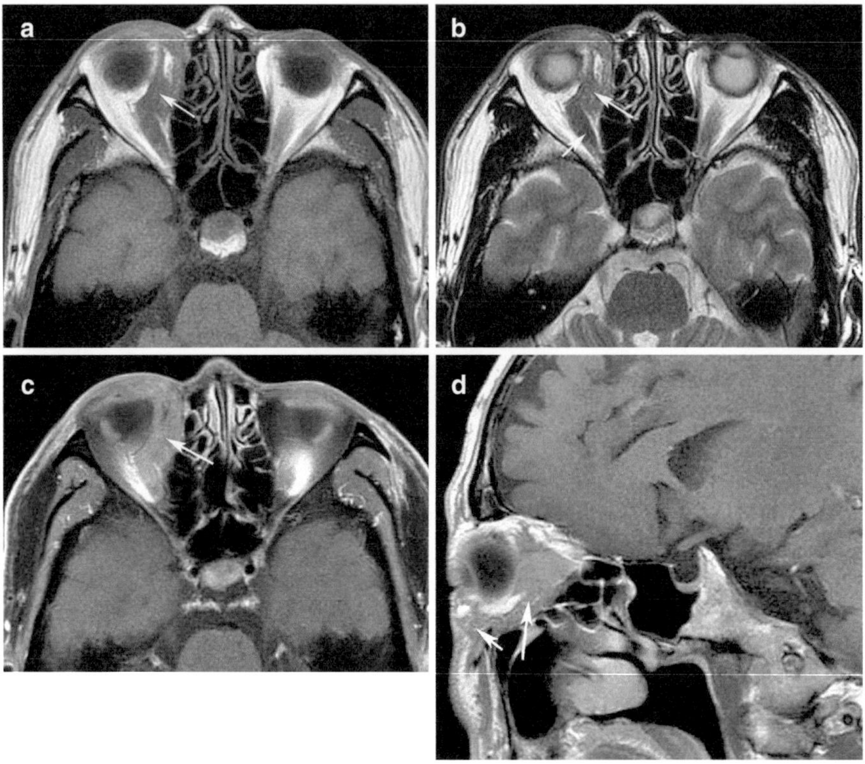

Fig. 5.3 Untypical lymphocyte hyperplasia. (**a**) Axial T1-weighted MR image shows an irregular lobulated isointense mass in the nasal side of the orbit (short white arrow). The mass extended anteriorly with eyelid and adjacent subcutaneous fat in the nasal dorsum involved, and posteriorly with intra- and extraconal space involved. The inferior rectus muscle including both tendon and venter is thickening. (**b**) Axial T2-weighted MR image shows the lesion isointense (long white arrow), and the inferior rectus muscle slightly hypointense (short white arrow). (**c**) Axial contrast-enhanced MR image shows the lesion with heterogeneous moderate enhancement. (**d**) Oblique sagittal contrast-enhanced MR image shows the preseptal structures are involved by the lesion and the eyelid and cheek soft tissue are thickening slightly (short white arrow). The eyeball is encased partially by the lesion and the inferior rectus muscle is involved, undistinguishable from the lesion

5.4 Evaluation

Ultrasound can display the lesion, but it is difficult to judge the relationship between the lesion and adjacent structures and to show the extent of involved structures outside the orbit. CT can show the extent of the lesion in the orbit and, furthermore, bone window can definitely show if there is bone change, but it is difficult to show the relationship between the lesion and adjacent structures. MRI can not only show the relationship between the lesion and adjacent structures but can also clearly show the extent of adjacent structures involved, including structures outside the orbit. Additionally, lymphoproliferative lesions can be differentiated from inflammatory pseudotumor according to signal intensity and enhancement pattern on MRI. Therefore, MRI is the best imaging technique for diagnosis of lymphoproliferative lesions (Akansel et al. 2005; Rojas Bilbao et al. 2010).

References

Akansel G, Hendrix L, Erickson BA, et al. MRI patterns in orbital malignant lymphoma and atypical lymphocytic infiltrates. Eur J Radiol. 2005;53(2):175–81.

Haradome K, Haradome H, Usui Y, et al. Orbital lymphoproliferative disorders (OLPDs): value of MR imaging for differentiating orbital lymphoma from benign OPLDs. AJNR. Am J Neuroradiol. 2014;35(10):1976–82.

Rojas Bilbao EA, Nesprias M, Pulero C, et al. Orbital and ocular adnexal lymphomas. Clinicopathological correlation in 25 cases. Medicina. 2010;70(4):333–8.

Talaulikar D, Tridgell D, Leong D, et al. Novel therapeutic option for orbital atypical lymphoid hyperplasia. Clin Exp Ophthalmol. 2010;38(9):892–4.

Chapter 6
Eyeball Diseases

Yongzhe Wang, Junfang Xian, and Zhengyu Zhang

6.1 Pigment Membrane Melanoma

6.1.1 Pathology

1. Malignant tumor with varying amounts of melanin arises from malignant transformation of the melanocytes or melanocytic nevi in uvea.
2. The tumor is composed of spindle-shaped A, B, or epithelial melanocytes (Sallam and Hungerford 2007).

6.1.2 Imaging Examination Recommendations

1. MRI is the first choice of examinations for pigment membrane melanoma and has an advantage to observe adjacent involved extent.
2. US can display the lesions, but its specificity significantly lower than that of MRI.
3. CT shows low sensitivity and specificity for the detection of smaller lesions.

Y. Wang • J. Xian (✉)
Department of Radiology, Beijing Tongren Hospital, Capital Medical University, Beijing, China
e-mail: cjr.xianjunfang@vip.163.com

Z. Zhang
Department of Radiology, Beijing Unicare ENT Hospital, Beijing, China

Z. Wang et al. (eds.), *Diagnostic Imaging of Ophthalmology*,
https://doi.org/10.1007/978-94-024-1060-0_6

6.1.3 Imaging Findings

MRI findings: The lesion in fusiform or mushroom-shaped appearance demonstrates homogenous hyperintensity on T1WI and homogenous hypointensity on T2WI, and strong enhancement after contrast injection (Figs. 6.1 and 6.2).

6.1.4 Conclusions

Pigment membrane melanoma is characterized by high signal on T1WI and low signal on T2WI in fusiform or mushroom-shaped appearance. It is not difficult for typical ones to differentiate from other lesions within the eyeball. The influence of the distribution and content of melanin on MR signal intensity may challenge the imaging diagnosis.

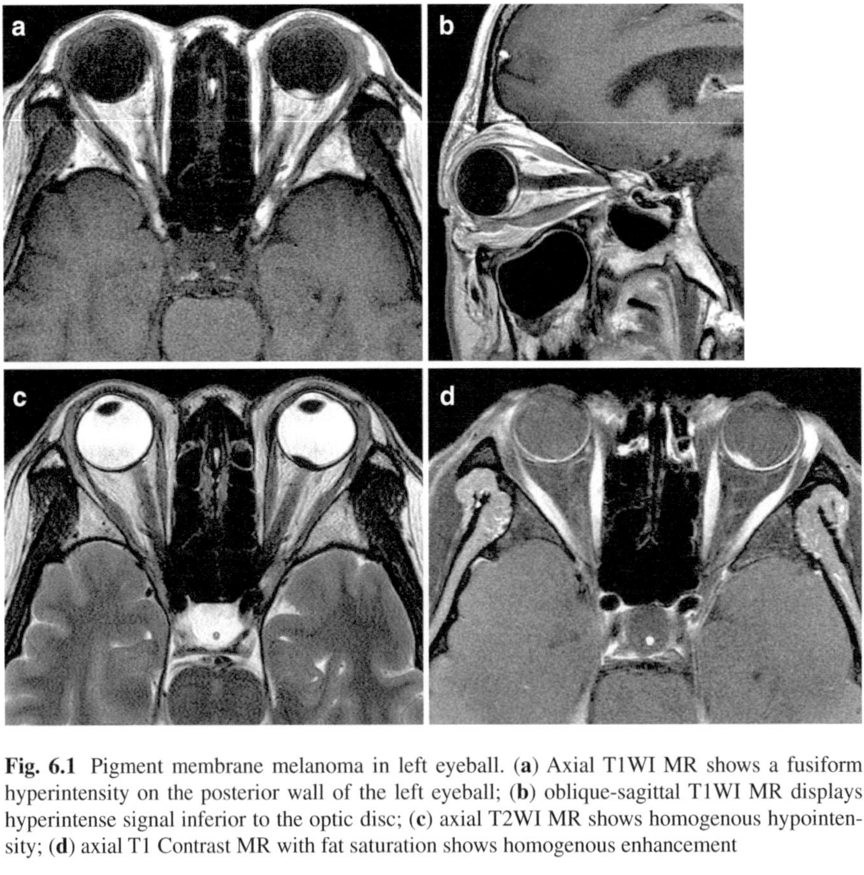

Fig. 6.1 Pigment membrane melanoma in left eyeball. (**a**) Axial T1WI MR shows a fusiform hyperintensity on the posterior wall of the left eyeball; (**b**) oblique-sagittal T1WI MR displays hyperintense signal inferior to the optic disc; (**c**) axial T2WI MR shows homogenous hypointensity; (**d**) axial T1 Contrast MR with fat saturation shows homogenous enhancement

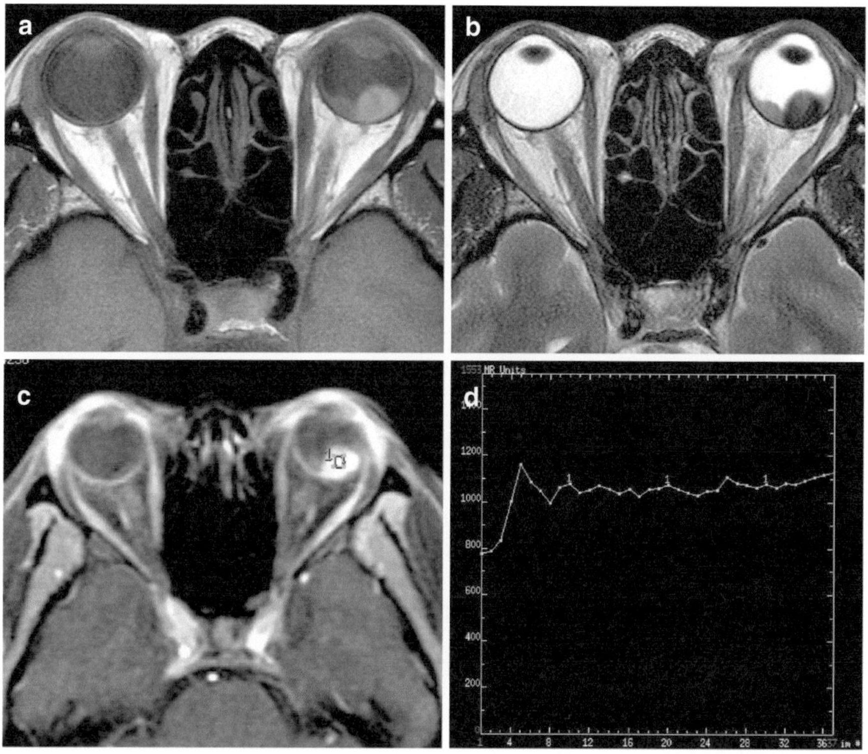

Fig. 6.2 Pigment membrane melanoma in left eyeball. (**a**) Axial T1WI MR shows hemispheric hyperintense signal on the posterior wall of the left eyeball; (**b**) axial T2WI MR displays homogenous low signal with retinal detachment; (**c**) the selection of ROI on DCE MRI; (**d**) the TIC on DCE MRI reveals enhancement within the lesion

6.2 Choroidal Hemangioma

6.2.1 Pathology

1. A benign, vascular hamartomatous lesion is actually cavernous hemangioma in most cases.
2. No pigment, round or oval orange or sallow flat lesion, often with retinal detachment.
3. Tumors are divided into two categories of solitary and diffusive one (Singh et al. 2005).

6.2.2 Imaging Examination Recommendations

1. US should be the first choice of examination due to its convenience.
2. MRI can become one of the preferred examination methods for those suspected cases difficult to diagnose.
3. CT has limited value due to its poor sensitivity and specificity.

6.2.3 Imaging Findings

MRI findings: The lesion shows fusiform or crescent appearance with well-definition and demonstrates homogenous iso-hypointense signal on T1WI and homogenous hyperintense signal on T2WI, and strong enhancement on contrast MRI (Figs. 6.3 and 6.4).

6.2.4 Conclusions

Ultrasound with the convenient and economic advantages is the first choice for this disease.It is difficult for CT to differentiate from other lesions such as choroid melanoma and metastases.MRI can clearly show the properties of the lesion and typical imaging characteristics.

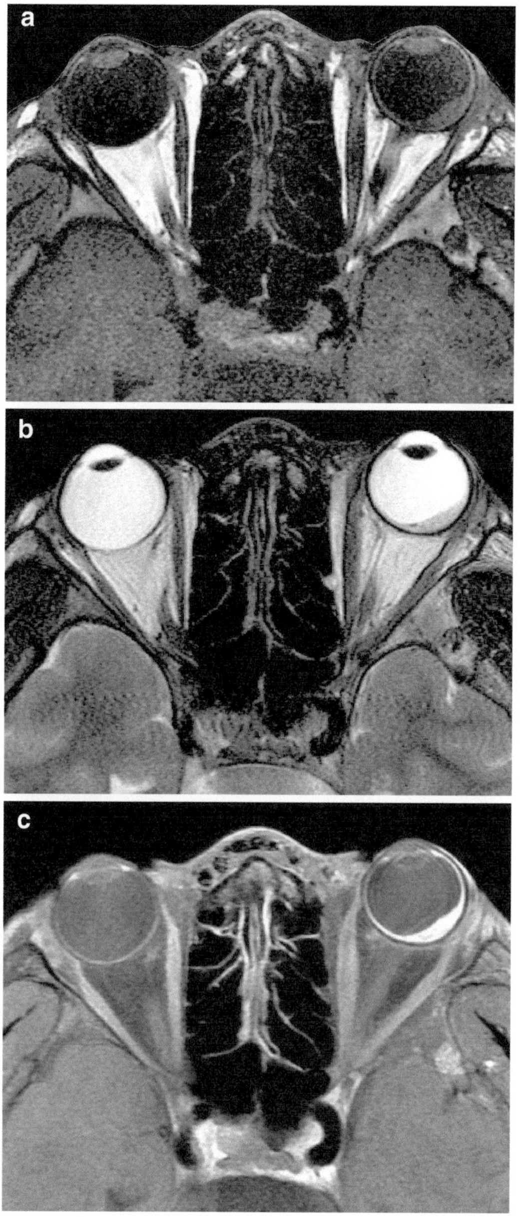

Fig. 6.3 Choroidal hemangioma in left eyeball. (**a**) Axial T1WI MR shows crescent isointense signal on the posterior wall of the left eyeball; (**b**) axial T2WI MR reveals homogenous hyperintense signal; (**c**) axial T1 Contrast MR with fat saturation shows homogenous significant enhancement

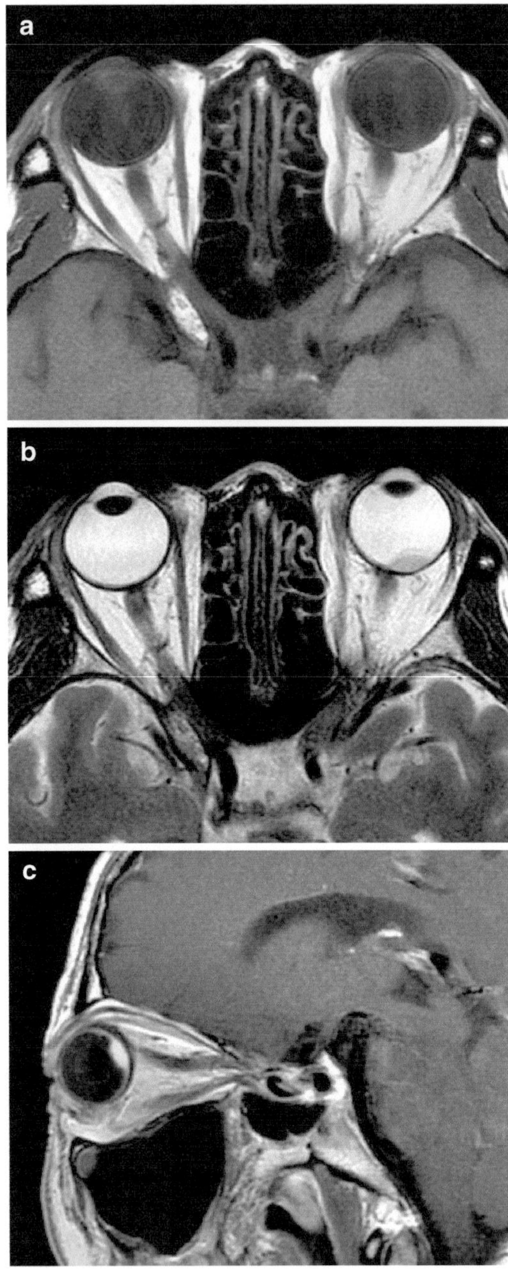

Fig. 6.4 Choroidal hemangioma in left eyeball. (**a**) Axial T1WI MR shows fusiform isointensity on the posterior wall of the left eyeball; (**b**) axial T2WI MR shows homogenous hyperintensity; (**c**) oblique-sagittal T1 Contrast MR demonstrates homogenous strong enhancement

6.3 Choroidal Osteoma

6.3.1 Pathology

1. Ophthalmoscope shows a white, elliptic, slightly elevated tumor, the uneven pigmentation in cluster is seen on the surface.
2. A benign tumor composed of mature bone tissue is usually flat or lenticular lens in appearance.

6.3.2 Imaging Examination Recommendations

1. CT is the first choice of examination because of higher sensitivity to bone tissue.
2. US becomes an important auxiliary examination means due to the simple, convenient advantages.
3. MRI is mainly used for those cases with the secondary retinal detachment.

6.3.3 Imaging Findings

1. CT findings: The lesion may occur in unilateral or bilateral eyeballs, a punctate, stripped, and curved high density located in the posterior wall of the eyeball (Fig. 6.5)

6.3.4 Conclusions

The confirmed diagnosis of choroidal osteoma can be made according to the characteristic CT manifestations.

Because of the low sensitivity to calcification and bone tissue, MRI is usually performed as a supplementary examination (Munteanu et al. 2008).

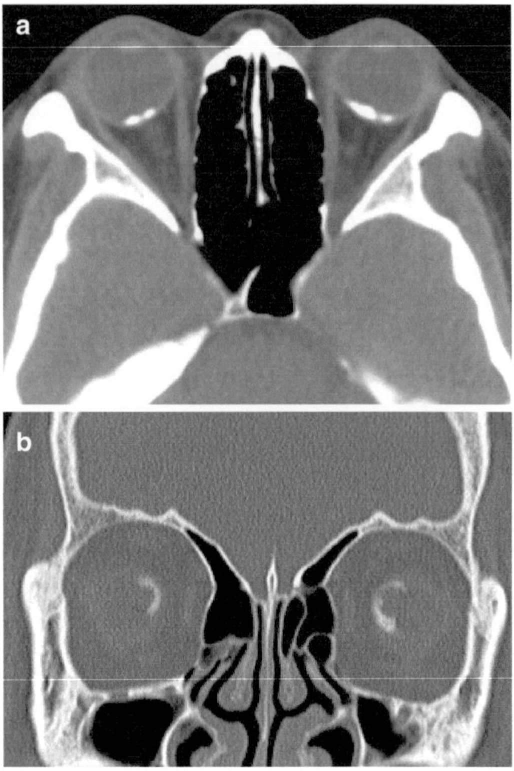

Fig. 6.5 (**a**) Axial soft tissue window CT shows punctate and stripped hyperdensity in posterior walls of bilateral eyeballs; (**b**) coronal bone window CT reveals curved high density

6.4 Choroidal Metastasis

6.4.1 Pathology

The tumor shows a flat mass in the color of yellow or no pigment on the fundus oculi. The secondary retinal detachment may occur (Arepalli et al. 2015).

6.4.2 Imaging Examination Recommendations

1. MRI is the first choice of examination.
2. The specificity of US is poor.
3. The smaller lesions may be difficultly found on CT.

6.4.3 Imaging Findings

MRI findings: The lesion with fusiform, crescent, or nodular appearance demonstrates isointense signal on T1WI, iso-hyperintense signal on T2WI, and marked enhancement on contrast enhanced MRI (Figs. 6.6 and 6.7).

6.4.4 Conclusions

The imaging features of choroidal metastasis have low specificity; it is suggestive of the diagnosis on the condition of primary tumor history. Otherwise, after eliminating melanoma, hemangioma or simple retinal detachment, choroidal metastasis should be taken into account.

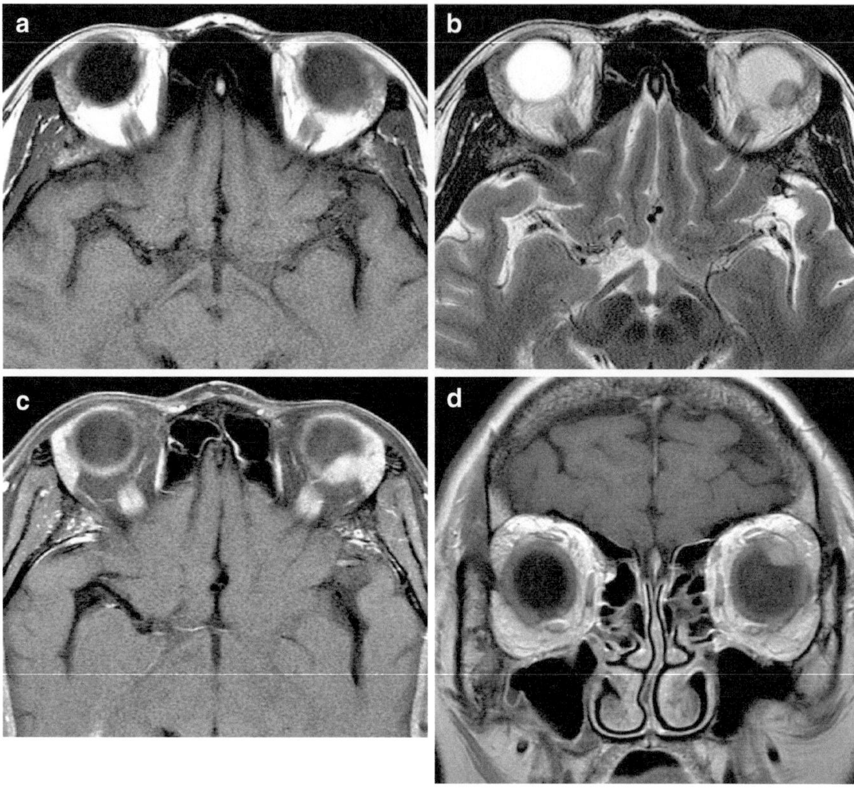

Fig. 6.6 Choroidal metastasis in left eyeball. (**a**) Axial T1WI MR shows fusiform isointense signal on the posterior wall of left eyeball; (**b**) axial T2WI MR reveals slightly hyperintense signal; (**c**) axial T1 Contrast MR with fat saturation displays homogenous significant enhancement; (**d**) coronal T1 Contrast MR demonstrate strongly enhanced mass on the superior-lateral wall of eyeball

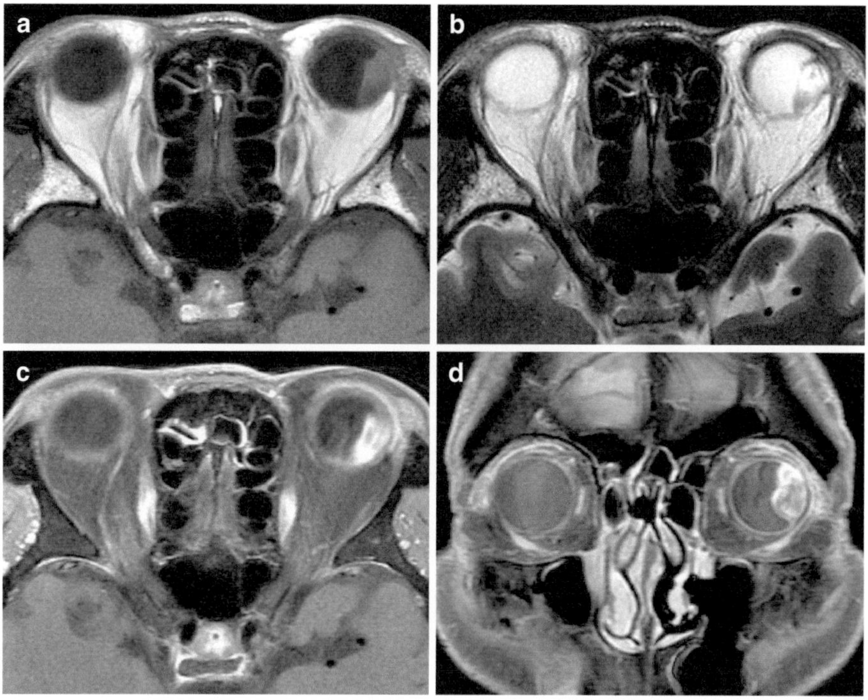

Fig. 6.7 Choroidal metastasis in left eyeball. (**a**) Axial T1WI MR shows fusiform hypointense signal on the lateral wall of left eyeball; (**b**) axial T2WI MR reveals heterogeneous hyperintense signal; (**c**) axial T1 Contrast MR with fat saturation displays heterogeneous significant enhancement. (**d**) coronal T1 Contrast MR with fat saturation demonstrates the lesion on the lateral wall of eyeball

6.5 Retinoblastoma

6.5.1 Pathology

1. The tumor originates from the retina with calcification and necrosis.
2. Histological features show undifferentiated neuroblasts with or without the coagulation necrosis.
3. The characteristic changes are the formation of the rosette of the tumor cells.
4. The calcinosis is common.

6.5.2 Imaging Examination Recommendations

1. CT is the first choice of examination due to the high sensitivity to the calcification.
2. MRI should be undergone for those patients suspected of the involvement of the extraocular and intracranial structures.
3. US can display the mass within the eyeball and is generally used for screening.

6.5.3 Imaging Findings

1. CT findings: The typical lesion displays soft tissue mass with punctate or patchy calcification in unilateral or bilateral eyeballs (Fig. 6.8).
2. MRI findings: The mass shows iso-hypointense signal on T1WI, isointense signal on T2WI and mild or significant enhancement on contrast enhanced MRI with or without retinal detachment (Figs. 6.9 and 6.10), (Rodriguez-Galindo et al. 2015).

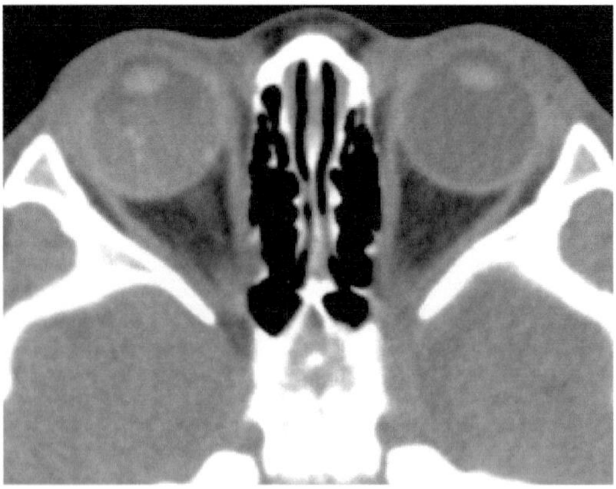

Fig. 6.8 Retinoblastoma in right eyeball. Axial soft tissue window CT shows an isodense mass with punctate calcification in right eyeball

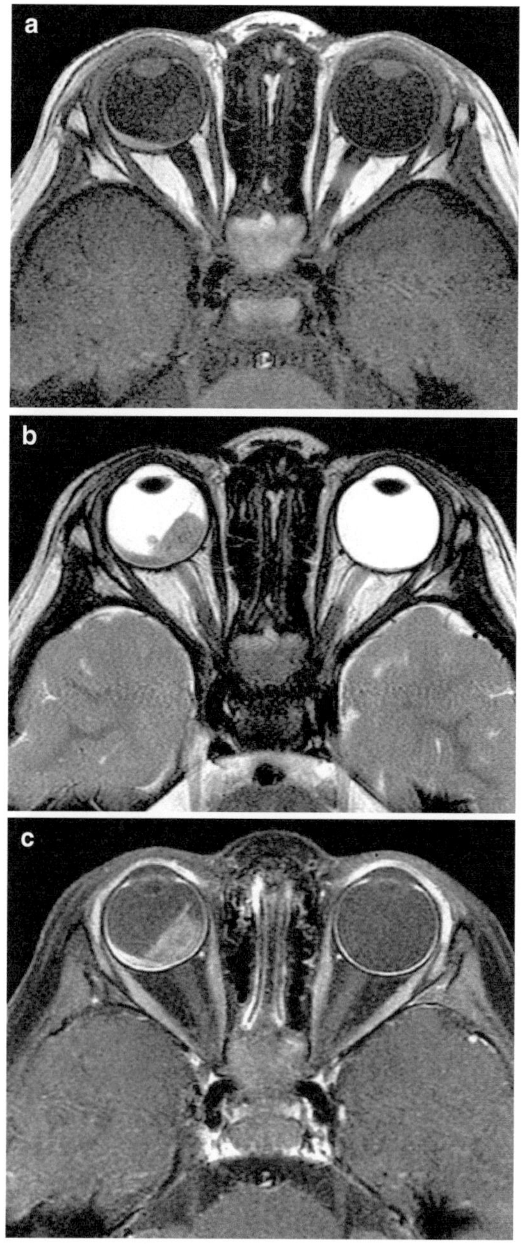

Fig. 6.9 Retinoblastoma in right eyeball with retinal detachment. (**a**) Axial T1WI MR shows hypointense signal in right eyeball with crescent high signal of retinal detachment; (**b**) axial T2WI MR reveals heterogeneous isointense signal of the mass and crescent isointense signal of retinal detachment; (**c**) axial T1 Contrast MR with fat saturation displays heterogenous mild enhancement

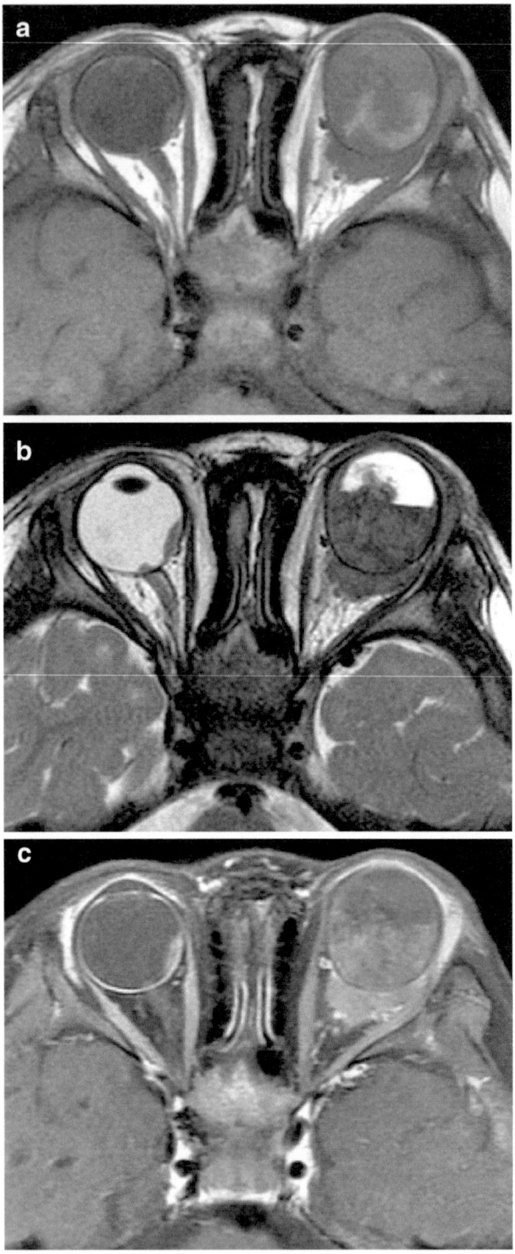

Fig. 6.10 Retinoblastoma in bilateral eyeballs with the extraocular involvement of the left lesion. (**a**) Axial T1WI MR shows heterogeneous iso-hyperintensity mass in left eyeball with the extraocular involvement and enlarged left eyeball and fusiform isointense signal on the intra-posterior wall in right eyeball; (**b**) axial T2WI MR reveals isointensity in bilateral eyeballs; (**c**) axial T1 Contrast MR with fat saturation displays heterogenous mild enhancement of the masses and shows the extent of the lesions clearly

6.5.4 Conclusions

The confirmed diagnosis is usually made according to the CT features and the predilection of below 3 years in children.

MRI can manifest the extent of the lesion and the involvement of the optic nerve and the intracranial structures.

6.6 Retinal Detachment

6.6.1 Pathology

1. The retinal neuroepithelium layer is separated from pigmentary epithelium layer.
2. According to the mechanism and etiology, the retinal detachment was divided into rhegmatogenous and nonrhegmatogenous one.
3. Rhegmatogenous retinal detachment is more common (Malbran 2007).

6.6.2 Imaging Examination Recommendations

1. US is the first choice for the method of the examination.
2. MRI should become one of the preferred examination methods for those cases with intraocular tumors.

6.6.3 Imaging Findings

MRI findings: The typical retinal detachment shows a "V" shape, tip at the optic disc and opening directing to ciliary body, detached retina can be seen, the signal of subretinal fluid varies with fluid compositions (Fig. 6.11).

6.6.4 Conclusions

Ultrasonic examination characterized by the convenient and economic advantages is the first choice for this disease. MRI should be performed for those cases secondary to intraocular tumors.

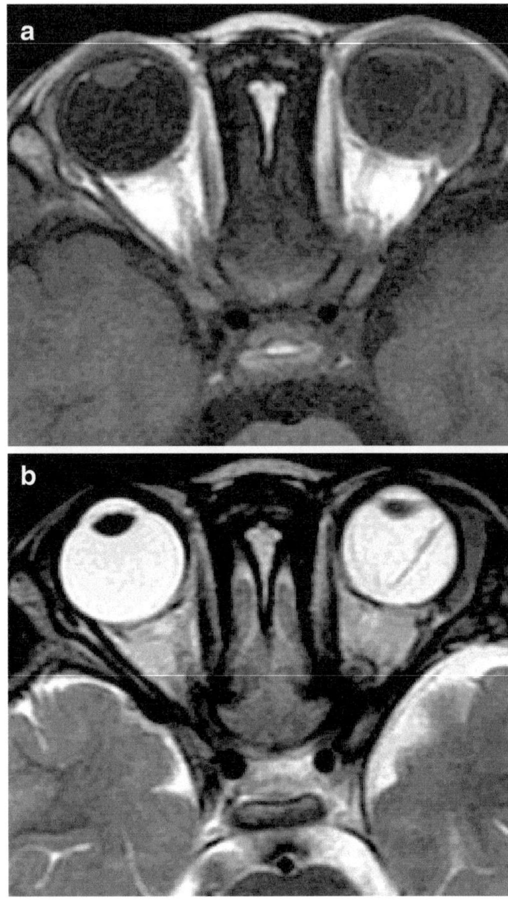

Fig. 6.11 Retinal detachment in left eyeball. (**a**) Axial T1WI MR shows slight hypointensity. (**b**) Axial T2WI MR reveals retinal detachment in "V" shape and hyperintensity of the subretinal dropsy

6.7 Phthisis Bulbi

The clinical terminology of the terminal period of eyeball destruction.

6.7.1 *Pathology*

1. Eyeball degeneration, eyeball atrophy, and calcification.
2. The destruction of intraocular structures resulted from severe ocular injury, endophthalmitis, multiple failed retinal detachment surgery, or extensive intraocular hemorrhage involving the ciliary body.
3. The state of retinoblastoma regression (Taha et al. 2015).

6.7.2 *Imaging Examination Recommendations*

1. US is the first choice of the examination methods.
2. CT can show the abnormal eyeball in shape and the calcification.

6.7.3 *Imaging Findings*

Us findings: The shrunken and deformed eyeball, the shortened eye axis, the widened, the disordered echo in vitreous body, the destroyed intraocular structures, and calcifications.

CT findings: An irregular shrunken eyeball with nodular calcification (Fig. 6.12).

6.7.4 *Conclusions*

Ultrasonic examination characterized by the convenient and economic advantages is the first choice for this disease. MRI should be performed for those cases secondary to intraocular tumors.

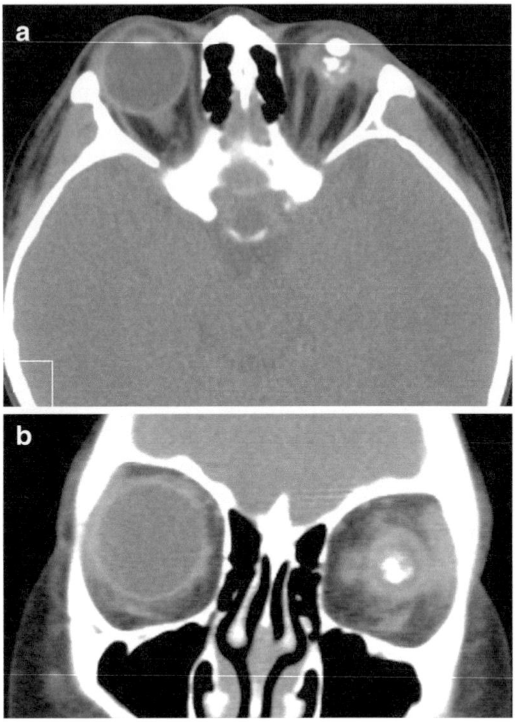

Fig. 6.12 Phthisis bulbi in left eyeball. (**a**) Axial soft tissue window CT shows an obviously shrunken left eyeball with nodular calcification; (**b**) coronal soft tissue window CT reveals an obviously shrunken left eyeball with nodular calcification

References

Arepalli S, Kaliki S, Shields CL. Choroidal metastases: origin, features, and therapy. Indian J Ophthalmol. 2015;63(2):122–7.

Malbran ES. Retinal detachment types. Ophthalmology. 2007;114(8):1591–2.

Munteanu M, Munteanu G, Zolog I, et al. Diffuse choroidal hemangioma associated with serous retinal detachment. Oftalmologia. 2008;52(2):59–63.

Rodriguez-Galindo C, Orbach C, Vanderveen C. Retinoblastoma. Pediatric Clin N Am. 2015;62(1):201–23.

Sallam A, Hungerford J. Choroidal melanoma. Br J Hosp Med. 2007;68(12):669–73.

Singh AD, Kaiser PK, Sears JE. Choroidal hemangioma. Ophthalmol Clin N Am. 2005;18(1):151–61.

Taha H, Amer HZ, El-Zomor H, et al. Phthisis bulbi: clinical and pathologic findings in retinoblastoma. Fetal Pediatric Pathol. 2015;34(3):176–84.

Chapter 7
Postoperative Change of Eyeball

Junfang Xian, Xinyan Wang, and Zhengyu Zhang

7.1 Post-Cataract Surgery

7.1.1 Pathology Features

1. Variable reasons such as aging, heredity, local malnutrition, immune and metabolism abnormalities, trauma, poisoning, and radiation all can cause metabolism disorders of crystalline lens, inducing degeneration of the lensprotein and lens turbidity, known as cataract.
2. The first choice of treatment for cataract is phacoemulsification combined with intraocular lens implantation. The ultrasound wave is used to comminute lens nucleus into chyle, which will be drawn off together with cortex. Posterior capsule of the lens is reserved for artificial lens embedding (Acharya et al. 2010).

7.1.2 Imaging Protocols

1. Usually, imaging is not needed for post-cataract surgery.
2. Postoperative change of cataract surgery is usually seen in old patients who perform imaging for other orbit lesion.

J. Xian (✉) • X. Wang
Department of Radiology, Beijing Tongren Hospital, Capital Medical University, Beijing, China
e-mail: cjr.xianjunfang@vip.163.com

Z. Zhang
Department of Radiology, Beijing Unicare ENT Hospital, Beijing, China

Z. Wang et al. (eds.), *Diagnostic Imaging of Ophthalmology*,
https://doi.org/10.1007/978-94-024-1060-0_7

7.1.3 Imaging Findings

1. MR imaging findings: A small strip showing isointense on T1WI and hypo-isointense on T2WI is found in the lens region with the normal lens absent (Fig. 7.1a).
2. CT findings: Nonenhanced CT imaging shows small strips with high density or slightly high density.

7.1.4 Evaluation

The normal lens is absent with a small strip in the corresponding region. The diagnosis and differential diagnosis is easy with consideration of medical history.

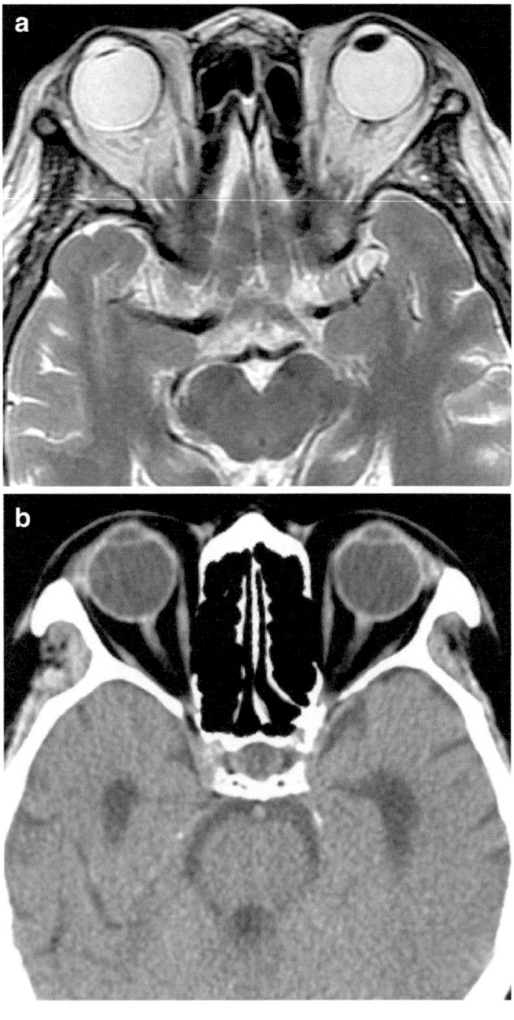

Fig. 7.1 Postoperative change of artificial lens implantation. (**a**) Axial T2-weighted MR image shows the normal lens of right side is absent with a small isointense strip found in the corresponding region; (**b**) axial nonenhanced CT image (another case) shows bilateral crystalline lenses are absent and small hyperdense strips are found in the corresponding regions

7.2 Postoperative Change of Vitrectomy

7.2.1 Pathology Features

1. Vitrectomy combined with gas or silicone oil tamponade is performed in patients for variable reasons such as complicated retinal detachment, vitreous hemorrhage, and macular diseases.
2. Cavum vitreum is usually filled with a small amount of fluid.

7.2.2 Imaging Protocols

1. Imaging is not necessary after vitreous body excision. If retinal detachment recurrence is suspected, fundus oculi cannot be observed due to turbidity of dioptric media or measurement of axis oculi is needed, ultrasound, MRI, or CT can be performed.
2. Ultrasound, as the first choice in clinical practice, is performed easily, but measurement of axis oculi is not accurate enough when cavum vitreum is filled with silicone oil.
3. MRI can demonstrate the postoperative change of vitrectomy and retinal detachment clearly. The accuracy of axis oculi measurement is not disturbed by silicone oil.
4. The role of CT is similar to that of MRI with disadvantage of radiation.

7.2.3 Imaging Findings

1. MRI findings: After vitrectomy combined with gas or silicone oil tamponade, the silicone oil filled in cavum vitreum shows high or slightly high signal intensity (Fig. 7.2a–c) on T1WI, high signal intensity on T2WI, and low or no signal intensity on fat saturation sequence (Fig. 7.2d), and no enhancement after contrast administration. In cases of vitrectomy combined with gas tamponade, the gas in cavum vitreum shows low signal intensity both on T1WI and T2WI.
2. CT findings: Silicone oil in the cavum vitreum displays as homogenous high density with 100 CT Hu. The fluid in the cavum vitreum is low or slightly low density, and the gas in the cavum vitreum is low density.

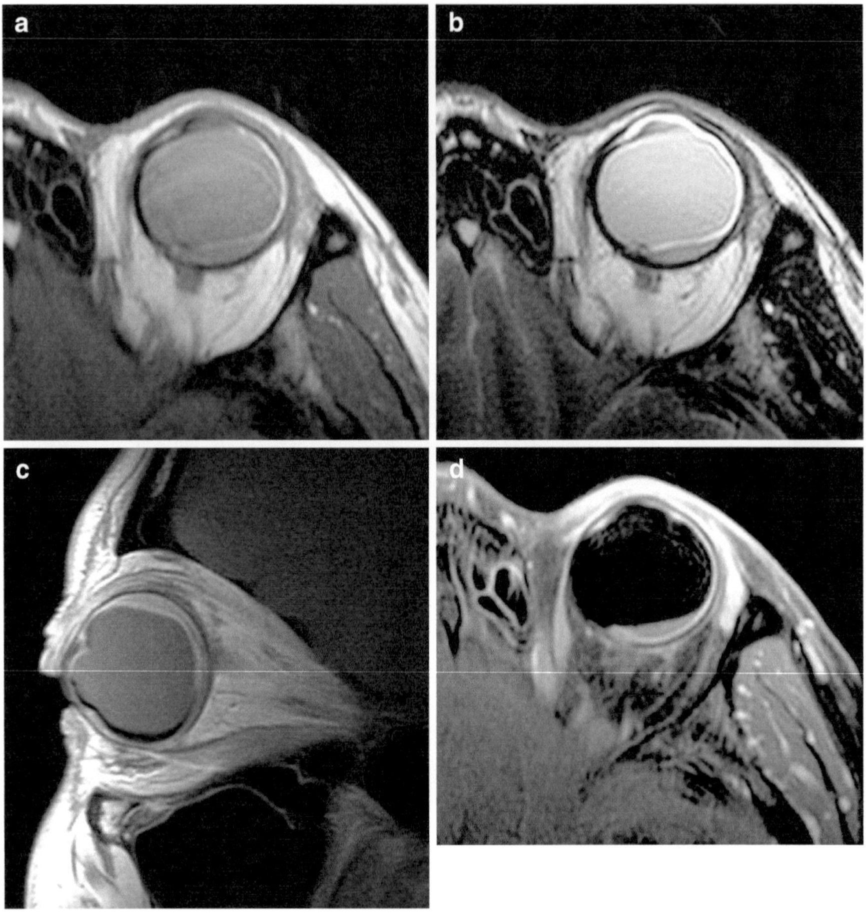

Fig. 7.2 Post-vitrectomy combined with silicone oil tamponade. (**a**) On axial T1-weighted MR image, the silicone oil in cavum vitreum shows homogeneous hyperintense signal with fluid-to-fluid level in posterior region. (**b**) On axial T2-weighted MR image, the silicone oil filled in cavum vitreum shows homogeneous high signal intensity with fluid-to-fluid level in the posterior area. (**c**) On oblique sagittal T1-weighted MR image, the silicone oil filled in cavum vitreum shows homogeneous high signal intensity with bracket-shaped hyperintense fluid accumulation in the upper posterior part and very low signal intensity of chemical shift artifacts in the inferior part. (**d**) On axial contrast T1-weighted MR image with fat saturation, the signal of silicone oil in the cavum vitreum is suppressed with fluid-to-fluid level in the posterior area

7.2.4 Evaluation

Postoperative change of vitreous body excision is easy to discriminate from other lesions due to its characteristic homogenous abnormal signal intensity in the vitreous body.

7.3 Section Postoperative Change of Scleral Buckling Surgery

7.3.1 Pathology Features

1. Scleral buckling is one of the common surgery treatments for rhegmatogenous retinal detachment. Pressurized material or buckle is put outside the sclera, which can compress the sclera to fit retinal neuroepithelium and pigment epithelium closely and to reduce the retina traction by vitreous body.
2. Surgical procedures include scleral explant buckling and scleral encircling operation, and the explant includes silicon sponge, elastic silica gel belt (2, 2. 5, and 4 mm wide), or cerebral dura mater (Ryan and Mittra 2010).

7.3.2 Imaging Protocols

1. Imaging is not necessary after scleral buckling. If retinal detachment recurrence is suspected, and fundus oculi cannot be observed due to turbidity of dioptric media, ultrasound, MRI, or CT can be performed.
2. Ultrasound can display the lesion, but its soft tissue resolution is lower than that of MRI.
3. MRI can definitely manifest the lesion.
4. The role of CT is similar to that of MRI with disadvantage of radiation.

7.3.3 Imaging Findings

1. CT findings: The anteroposterior diameter of eyeball is enlarged with Hourglass sign. Scleral buckles usually manifest as bands near the equator and encircling the eyeball. Silica gel belt manifests as hyperdense small strip on axial image, and circular high density encircling the scleral on oblique coronal image, which is well defined and regular (Fig. 7.3a–c).
2. MRI findings: The morphology demonstrated on MRI is similar to that on CT. Scleral buckle is hypointense on T1WI and T2WI (Fig. 7.3d).

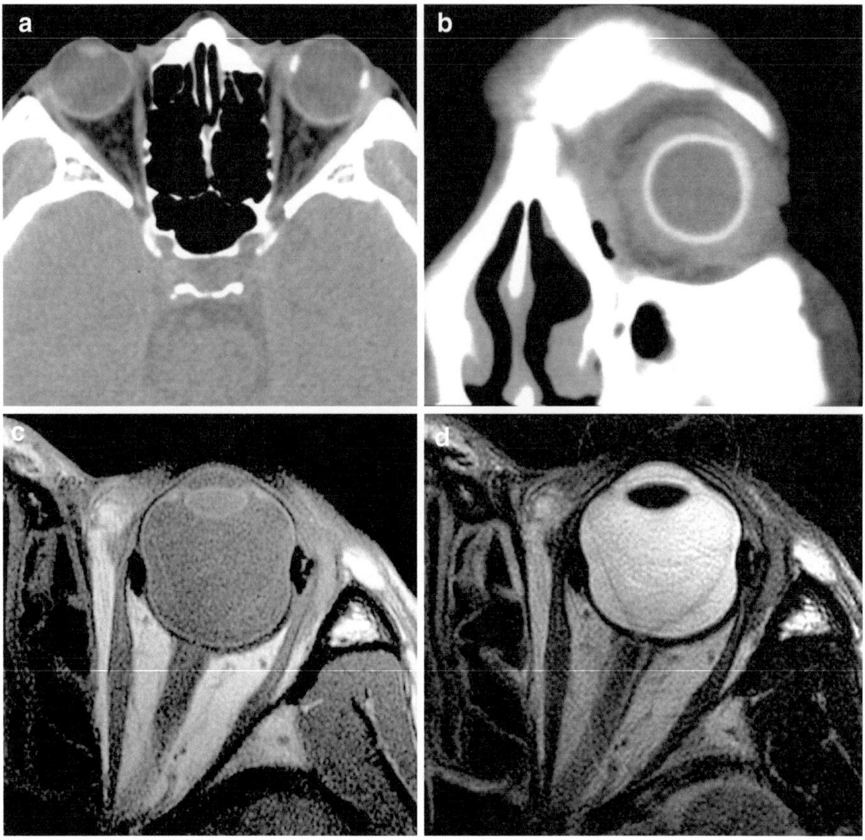

Fig. 7.3 Postoperative change of scleral buckling surgery. (**a**) Nonenhanced axial CT image shows the anteroposterior diameter of the left eyeball is enlarged, and symmetrical hyperdense strips are found in the equator region; (**b**) nonenhanced oblique coronal CT image manifest scleral buckles as circular high density in the equator of eyeball; (**c**) on axial T1-weighted MR image, the scleral buckle shows as symmetrical hypointense strips. V-shaped low signal intensity is found pointing to optic disc, which indicates retinal detachment; (**d**) on axial T2-weighted MR image, the scleral buckle shows as symmetrical hypointense strips. V-shaped high signal intensity indicating retinal detachment can be seen pointing to optic disc

7.4 Postoperative Change of Enucleation

7.4.1 Pathology Features

1. Based on complete loss of vision, eyeball enucleation is performed in order to relieve megalgia of the affected eye, to remove threats to the healthy eye, to prevent malignant tumors spread which may threaten one's life, or to improve one's appearance hindered by the affected eye.
2. Eye enucleation is classified into simple eye enucleation and orbital buried implantation after enucleation. In simple eye enucleation, superior and inferior rectus muscles and lateral and medial rectus muscles are ligatured, respectively, into a cross shape without materials implantation. In orbital buried implantation after enucleation, the four rectus muscles are sutured in the corresponding site on the implant.
3. Generally, implants buried after enucleation include biological material and synthetic material. Biological materials include self-tissue, allogenic tissue, and heteroplasm, and synthetic materials include metals, biological ceramic (hydroxyapatite) and polymer, etc. At present, hydroxyapatite is the best orbit filling material, most of which is round or ellipse ocular prosthesis with diameter of 16–24 mm. After implantation, surrounding blood vessels grow into the artificial eyeball soon, and osteocytes are deposited onto its surface which grow into the micropore of the implant continually and centripetally. The ossification and vascularization of the artificial eyeball make itself as one part of the body and will not be removed (Steeves and Gonzalez 2008).

7.4.2 Imaging Protocols

1. Usually, image examination after enucleation is performed to exclude malignant tumor recurrence or metastasis.
2. Ultrasound can display the lesion, but its soft tissue resolution is lower than that of MRI.
3. MRI is the best imaging method which can demonstrate the extent and characteristic of the lesion.
4. CT is not as good as MRI for characterization of the lesion.

7.4.3 Imaging Findings

1. CT findings: The normal eyeball is absent, and extraocular muscles and optic nerve get shorter and thinner. Global heterogeneous high density is found in the anterior part of the orbit after hydroxyapatite sphere implantation, which is well

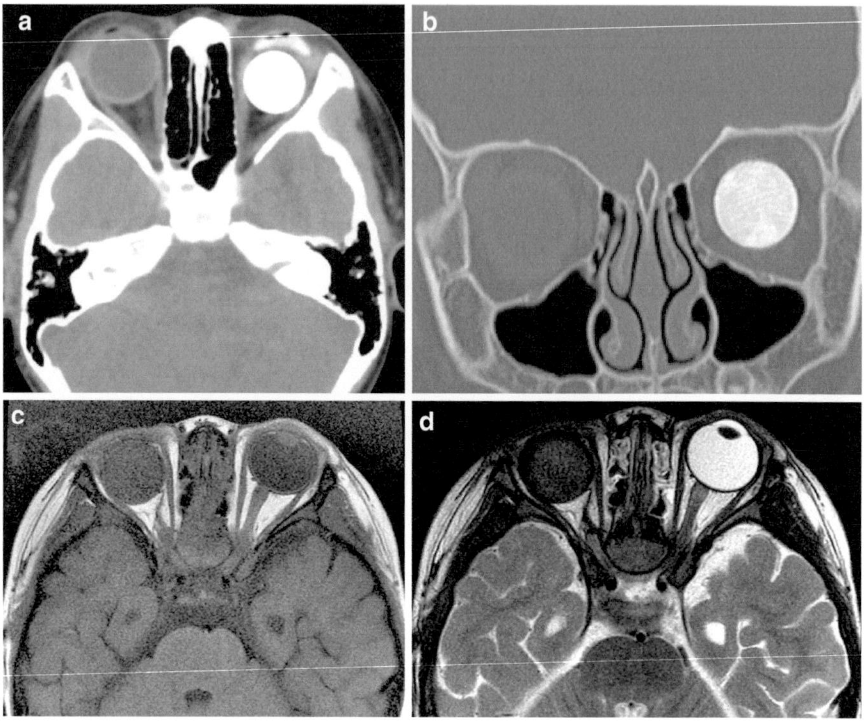

Fig. 7.4 Post hydroxyapatite sphere implantation after enucleation of eyeball. (**a**) Cross-sectional CT soft tissue window shows a rounded high-attenuation area (the hydroxyapatite sphere implantation) in the anterior part of the left orbit, in front of which is an arc-shaped high density indicating the ocular prosthesis. (**b**) Coronal-sectional CT bone window of the same patient shows well defined quasi-circular heterogeneous high density in the anterior part of the left orbit. (**c**) Cross-sectional T1-weighted MRI reveals that the right normal eyeball is absent and instead there is a well-defined circular slightly hypointense area in the corresponding location with no display of intraorbital optic nerve. (**d**) Cross-sectional T2-weighted MRI of the same patient shows well-defined circular heterogeneous slightly hypointense in the anterior part of the right orbit

defined and attached with extraocular muscles. Ocular prosthesis can be or not be found anterior to hydroxyapatite sphere (Fig. 7.4a, b).

2. MRI findings: Hydroxyapatite orbital implantation shows heterogeneous isointense or slightly hypointense on T1WI, and heterogeneous isointense or slightly hyperintense on T2WI with grid appearance. When blood vessels grow inwards, the orbital implantation shows enhancement after contrast administration.

References

Acharya RU, Yu W, Zhu K, et al. Identification of cataract and post-cataract surgery optical images using artificial intelligence techniques. J Med Syst. 2010;34(4):619–28.
Ryan EH, Mittra RA. Scleral buckling vs vitrectomy: the continued role for scleral buckling in the vitrectomy era. Arch Ophthalmol. 2010;128(9):1202–5.
Steeves JKE, Gonzalez EG, Steinbach MJ. Vision with one eye: a review of visual function following unilateral enucleation. Spat Vis. 2008;21(6):509.

Chapter 8
Orbital Vasogenic Diseases

Junfang Xian, Yongzhe Wang, and Zhengyu Zhang

8.1 Cavernous Hemangioma

8.1.1 Pathology

1. A round, oval, or lobulated mass in dark purple with a thin fibrous capsule.
2. Actually, the venous malformation, rather than a true tumor, is made up of different vascular sinuses in size and shape. The section shows cavernous, porous in appearance and fiber separation among vascular cavities.

8.1.2 Imaging Examination Recommendations

1. CT is the first choice of examination for the clinical suspected lesions posterior to eyeball.
2. MRI: an essential examination method for confirming the properties of the mass and the involved adjacent structures.

J. Xian (✉) • Y. Wang
Department of Radiology, Beijing Tongren Hospital, Capital Medical University, Beijing, China
e-mail: cjr.xianjunfang@vip.163.com

Z. Zhang
Department of Radiology, Beijing Unicare ENT Hospital, Beijing, China

Z. Wang et al. (eds.), *Diagnostic Imaging of Ophthalmology*,
https://doi.org/10.1007/978-94-024-1060-0_8

8.1.3 Imaging Findings

1. CT findings: An oval or round mass in intraconal space with well-circumstance shows isodensity, with punctate calcification in minority cases.
2. MRI findings: The lesion displays homogeneous hypointense signal on T1WI, homogeneous hyperintensity on T2WI, and marked enhancement on contrast enhanced MRI. The hypointensity of fiber septation can be found on T2WI. Peripheral hypointensity chemical shift artifact is also seen. The typical feature of progressive enhancement is seen on DCE MRI, the TIC shows a steady enhancement pattern (Figs. 8.1 and 8.2) (Ansari and Mafee 2005; Dallaudiere et al. 2009).

8.1.4 Conclusions

Cavernous hemangioma shows soft tissue density on CT and difficultly differentiates with other tumors in orbital cavity.

MRI can show the relationship of lesion with the adjacent structures, according to the characteristic of "progressive enhancement" on DCE MRI; it is not difficult to differentiate from other tumors in intraconal space.

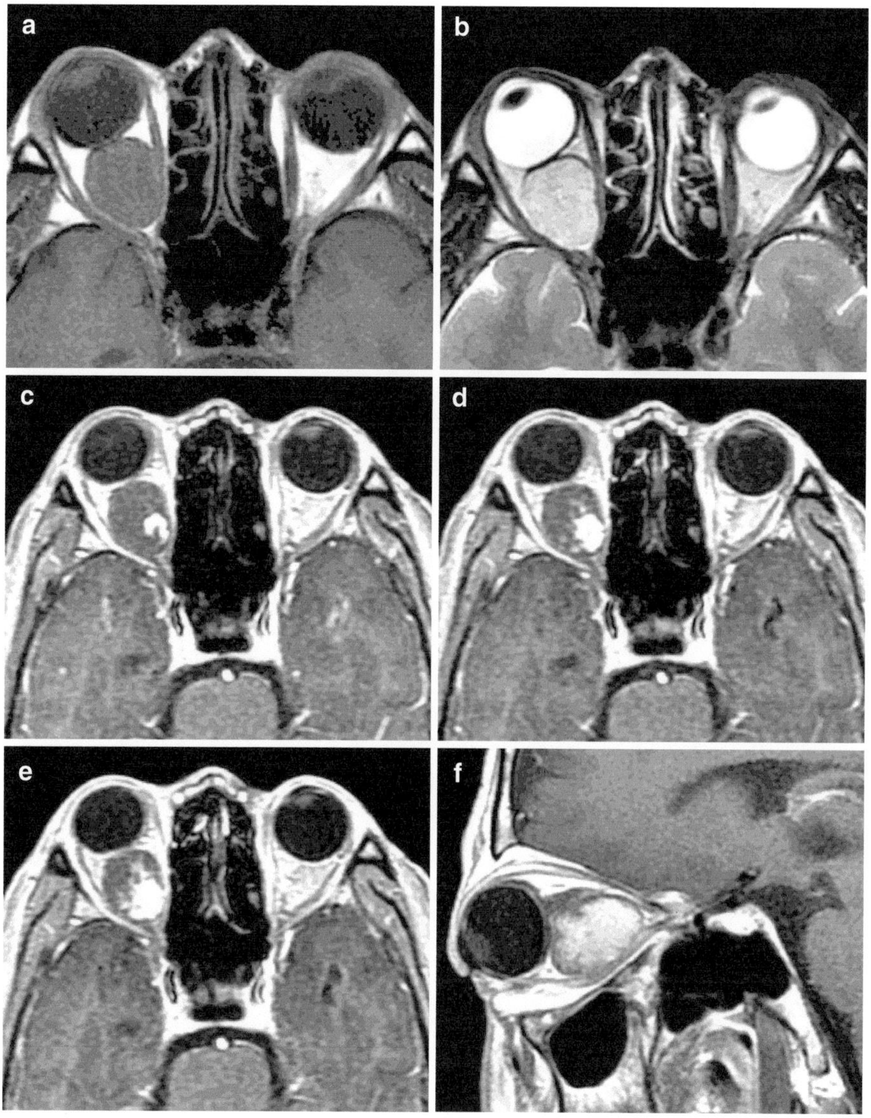

Fig. 8.1 Cavernous hemangioma in right orbit. (**a**) Axial T1WI MR shows oval homogeneous low intensity in right intraconal space; (**b**) axial T2WI MR reveals homogeneous hyperintense signal; (**c**) axial DCE MR shows patchy enhancement within the lesion; (**d**) axial DCE MR shows that the area of patchy enhancement is bigger than that of (**c**); (**e**) axial DCE MR shows that the area of patchy enhancement is bigger than that of (**d**); (**f**) oblique-sagittal T1Contrast MR demonstrates homogeneous significant enhancement

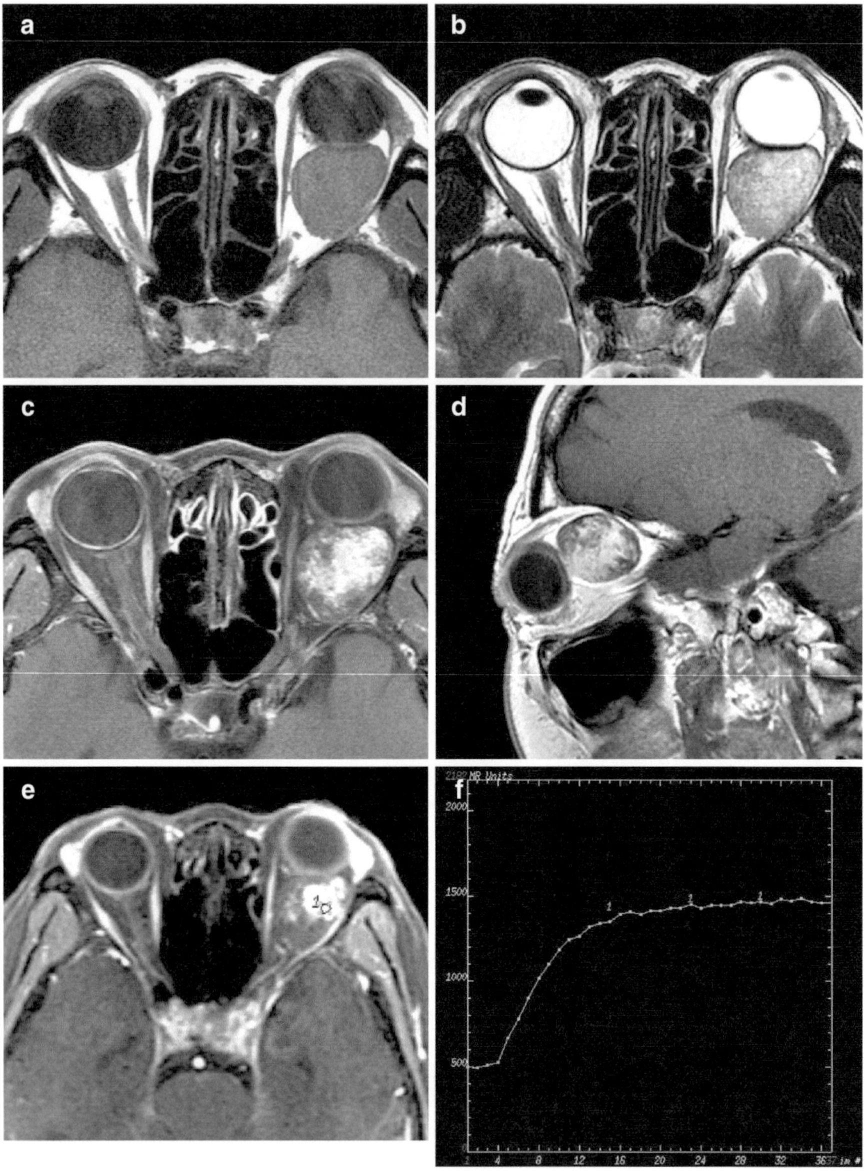

Fig. 8.2 Cavernous hemangioma in left orbit. (**a**) Axial T1WI MR shows oval homogeneous isointensity in left intraconal space; (**b**) axial T2WI MR reveals homogeneous hyperintense signal; (**c**) axial T1Contrast MR with fat saturation shows strong patchy enhancement within the lesion; (**d**) oblique-sagittalT1Contrast MR demonstrates a mass between the superior rectus and the optic nerve; (**e**) axial DCE MR shows that the selection of ROI; (**f**) the TIC on DCE MR shows a steady enhancement pattern

8.2 Lymphangioma

8.2.1 Pathology

1. An irregular mass without capsule composed of lymphatic vessels in different sizes.
2. The lesion is mainly composed of pipelines lining transparent endothelial cells containing serosity and myxoid matrix composition. Old or fresh blood, lymphocyte accumulation, and small vascular dysplasia are also seen (Héran et al. 2014).

8.2.2 Imaging Examination Recommendations

1. CT is the first choice of examination for the clinical suspected lesions.
2. MRI should be undergone to manifest the properties of mass and the relationship with the adjacent structures.

8.2.3 Imaging Findings

CT findings: An irregular or diffusive mass in shape shows heterogeneous iso-hypodensity with or without punctate vein stone; the high density like fluid-fluid level can be found within the lesion if fresh hemorrhage occurs.

MRI findings: The lesion displays heterogeneous intense signal with typical fluid-fluid level due to the hemorrhage in different periods and heterogeneous slight or mild enhancement (Figs. 8.3 and 8.4).

8.2.4 Conclusions

On CT, the lymphangioma shows a soft tissue density in irregular shape; it is difficult for the diffusive lesions to differentiate from other orbital tumors such as varix.

MRI can clearly demonstrate the signal features within the lesions, the characteristic fluid-fluid level, and the relationship with adjacent structures; it is helpful to differentiate from other orbital tumors.

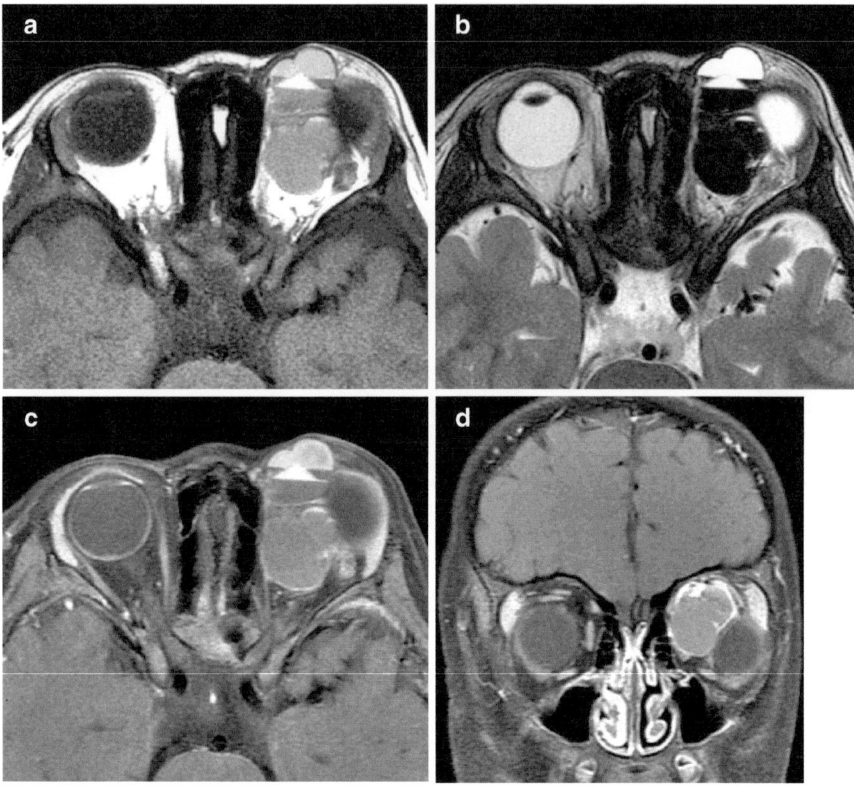

Fig. 8.3 Local lymphangioma in left orbit. (**a**) Axial T1WI MR shows heterogeneous intensity in irregular shape with fluid-fluid level in left orbit; (**b**) axial T2WI MR reveals heterogeneous signal with fluid-fluid level; (**c**) axial T1Contrast MR with fat saturation shows slight peripheral enhancement; (**d**) coronal T1Contrast MR with fat saturation demonstrates the mass in the superomedial region of the left orbit

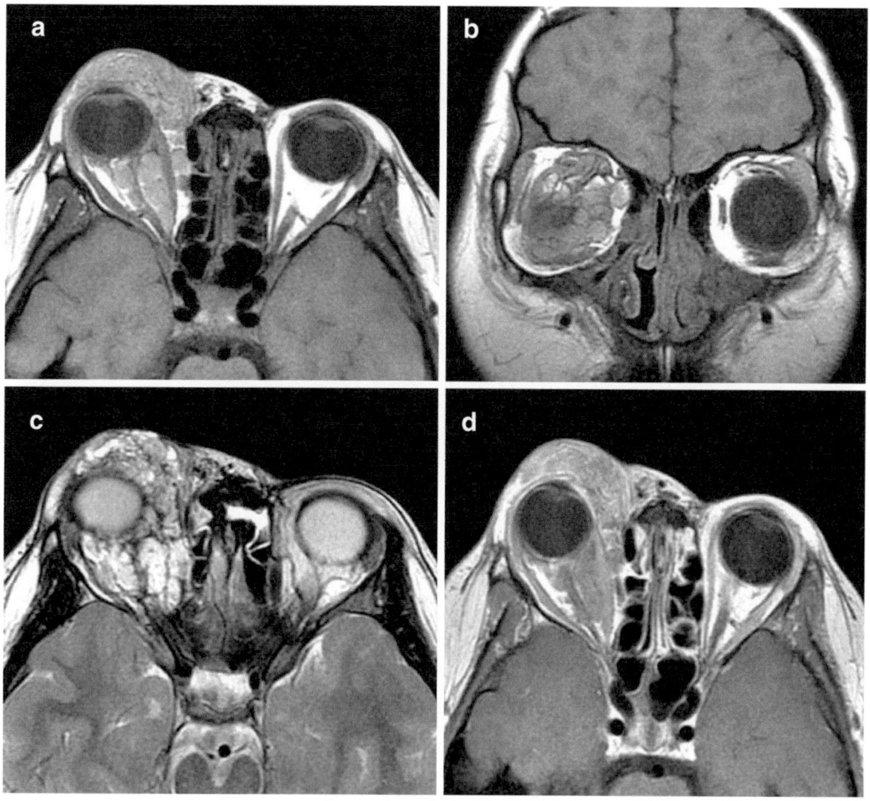

Fig. 8.4 Diffusive lymphangioma in right orbit. (**a**) Axial T1WI MR shows isointense signal in irregular shape with the diffusive involvement of the right intra-extraconal space; (**b**) coronalT1WI MR reveals ill-circumstance with the adjacent optic nerve and extraocular muscles; (**c**) axial T2WI MR shows heterogeneous hyperintensity with hypointense septa; (**d**) axial T1Contrast MR shows heterogeneous slight enhancement

8.3 Capillary Angioma

8.3.1 Pathology

1. The tumor has no capsule; the gray parenchyma of the tumor is in granular appearance and is fragile.
2. The tumor is composed of vascular endothelial cells and capillaries. In the period of tumor regression, due to capillary atresia, blood vessels are replaced by fat, and the tumor can completely become fat and fibrosis finally.

8.3.2 Imaging Examination Recommendations

Both of CT and MRI can determine the extent of capillary angioma, T1WI or T1Contrast MR with fat saturation are superior to other sequences.

8.3.3 Imaging Findings

1. CT findings: The lesion usually occurs in eyelid or pre-septal space and shows an irregular soft tissue density with or without the involvement of post-septal space.
2. MRI findings: The lesion displays iso-hypointense signal on T1WI, homogeneous hyperintensity on T2WI, and heterogeneous slight or marked enhancement on contrast enhanced MRI (Fig. 8.5).

8.3.4 Conclusions

The diagnosis of capillary hemangioma is confirmed easily in clinic. The objective of CT and MRI examination is to determine the involved extent of the lesion, and MRI is superior to CT on this aspect.

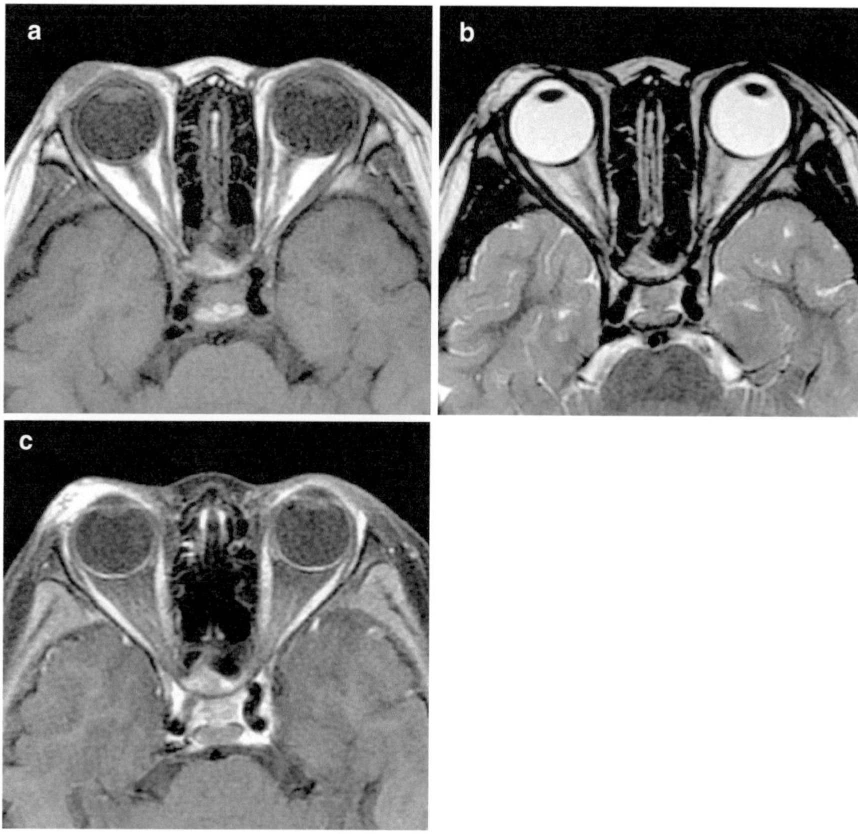

Fig. 8.5 Capillary angioma in right eyelid. (**a**) Axial T1WI MR shows homogeneous isointense signal in right eyelid; (**b**) axial T2WI MR reveals homogeneous hyperintense signal; (**c**) axial T1Contrast MR with fat saturation shows heterogeneous strong enhancement

8.4 Varix

8.4.1 Pathology

1. Varix is actually some incomplete vascular tissues with large vascular cavity, thin wall and loose vascular endothelial cells, and smooth muscle fibers; there are many intraluminal thromboses. A certain amount of fibrous tissues exist among the blood vessels with inflammatory cell infiltration.
2. Lack of the inner elastic layer and the elastic fiber tissue in the vascular wall, the input and the output blood vessels are all veins.

8.4.2 Imaging Examination Recommendations

For those patients with positional exophthalmos, MRI, CT, or US is performed after compressing neck vessels or changing position.

8.4.3 Imaging Findings

CT findings: The lesion shows isodensity with ill-definition in irregular shape.

MRI findings: The lesion reveals iso-hypointense on T1WI, hyperintense on T2WI, and slow strong enhancement on contrast enhanced MRI. The enlarged mass is seen after compressing neck vessels. If thrombosis occurs within the lesion, non-enhanced area is found (Figs. 8.6 and 8.7) (White et al. 2005).

8.4.4 Conclusions

The diagnosis of varix can be confirmed according to a significantly enlarged lesion on imaging examination after compression on neck or positional changes.

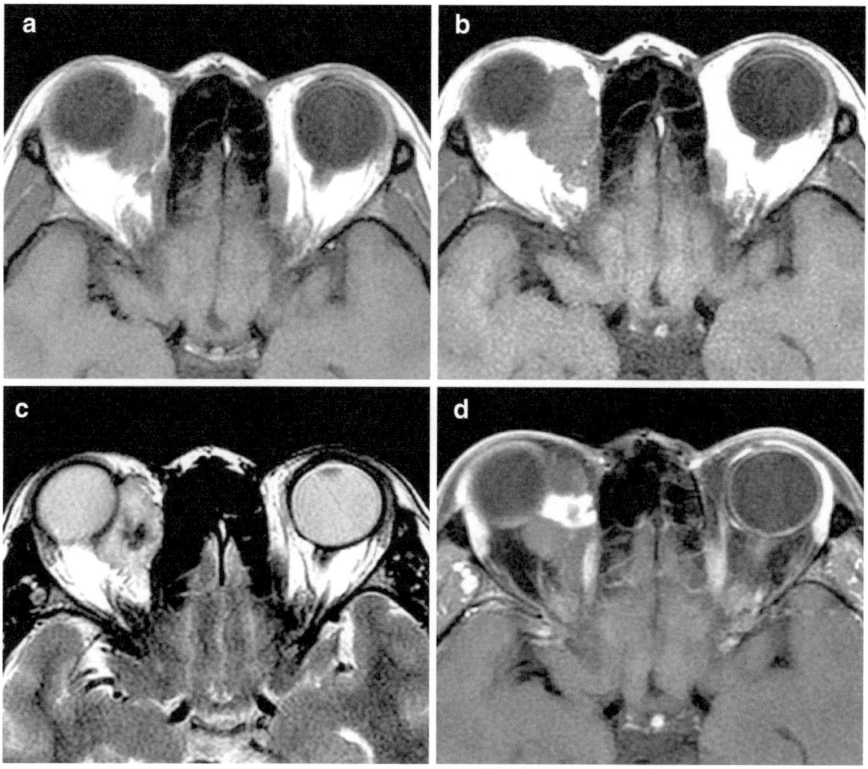

Fig. 8.6 Varix in right orbit. (**a**) Axial T1WI MR (before compression on neck vessels) shows isointensity in irregular shape in right orbit; (**b**) axial T1WI MR (after compression on neck vessels) reveals the lesion enlarged significantly; (**c**) axial T2WI MR (after compression on neck vessels) shows hyperintense signal with patchy low signal; (**d**) axial T1Contrast MR with fat saturation (after compression on neck vessels) shows patchy strong enhancement within the lesion

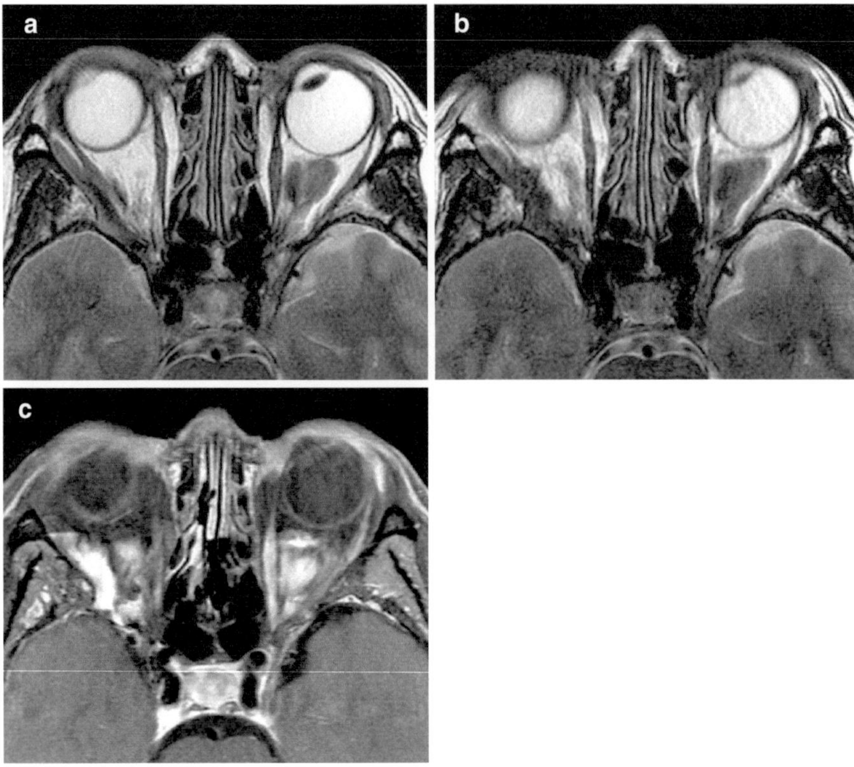

Fig. 8.7 Varix in bilateral orbits. (**a**) Axial T2WI MR (before compression on neck vessels) shows isointensity in irregular shape in bilateral orbits; (**b**) axialT2WI MR (after compression on neck vessels) reveals the extent of lesions enlarged; (**c**) axial T1Contrast MR with fat saturation (after compression on neck vessels) demonstrates marked enhancement in involved areas

8.5 Carotid Cavernous Fistula

8.5.1 *Pathology*

1. The ruptured cavernous sinus segment of internal carotid artery or small branches lead to an abnormal arteriovenous communication with cavernous sinus.
2. Over 75% of cases are resulted from injury; spontaneous cases are also seen (Chaudhry et al. 2009).

8.5.2 *Imaging Examination Recommendations*

1. CT is the first choice of examination for the clinically suspected CCF on the condition of eye injury. CTA and MRA are also performed further.
2. MRI is used as a supplementary examination method.

8.5.3 *Imaging Findings*

CT and MRI findings: Proptosis, enlarged superior ophthalmic vein, enlarged cavernous sinus, blurry intra-extraconal space, enlarged extraocular muscle, eyelid swelling. CTA and MRA can show the abovementioned findings and abnormal draining veins and fistula in some cases (Figs. 8.8 and 8.9) (Venkataramaiah and Sriganesh 2014).

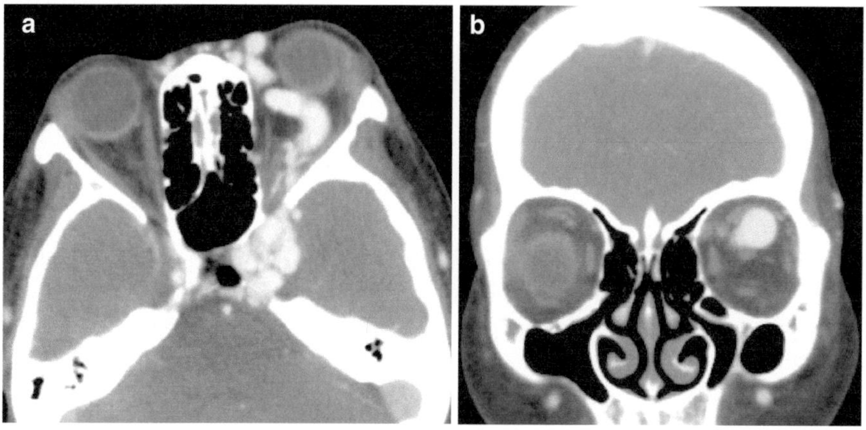

Fig. 8.8 Carotid cavernous fistula in left orbit. (**a**) Axial enhanced CT shows enlarged cavernous sinus, superior ophthalmic vein and the tortuous vessels in inner canthus; (**b**) coronal enhanced CT reveals enlarged superior ocular vein

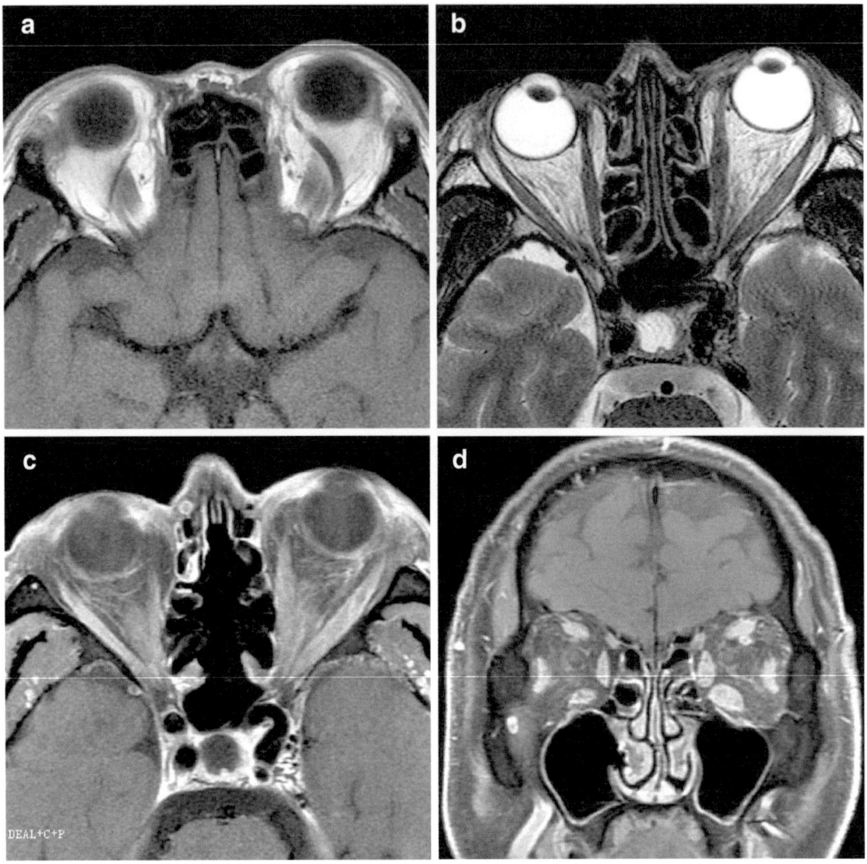

Fig. 8.9 Carotid cavernous fistula in left orbit. (**a**) Axial T1WI MR shows enlarged superior ocular vein; (**b**) axialT2WI MR reveals enlarged extraocular muscles; (**c**) axial T1Contrast MR with fat saturation shows multiple small vessels in left enlarged cavernous sinus, blurry intra-extraconal space, eyelid swelling; (**d**) coronal T1Contrast MR with fat saturation demonstrates enlarged extraocular muscles

8.5.4 Conclusions

Combined with clinical history, carotid cavernous fistula should be taken into account according to enlarged superior ocular vein and cavernous fistula on CT and MRI. DSA is still the golden standard for the confirmed diagnosis of carotid cavernous fistula.

References

Ansari SA, Mafee MF. Orbital cavernous hemangioma: role of imaging. Neuroimaging Clin N Am. 2005;15(1):137–58.

Chaudhry IA, Elkhamry SM, Al-Rashed W, et al. Carotid cavernous fistula: ophthalmological implications. Middle East African J Ophthal. 2009;16(2):57–63.

Dallaudiere B, Benayoun Y, Boncoeur-Martel M, et al. Imaging features of cavernous hemangiomas of the orbit. J Radiol. 2009;90(9):1039–45.

Héran F, Bergès O, Blustajn J, et al. Tumor pathology of the orbit. Diagn Interv Imaging. 2014;95(10):933–44.

Venkataramaiah S, Sriganesh K. Images in clinical medicine. Carotid cavernous fistula. N Engl J Med. 2014;371(19):1832.

White JH, Fox AJ, Symons SP. Diagnosis and anatomic mapping of an orbital varix by computed tomographic angiography. Am J Ophthalmol. 2005;140(5):945–7.

Chapter 9
Orbital Tumor

Dapeng Hao, Zhenchang Wang, and Zhengyu Zhang

9.1 Schwannoma

9.1.1 Pathology

1. The tumor is well defined, encapsulated, ovoid, or fusiform.
2. Cystic degeneration and hemorrhage are commonly seen in the tumor.
3. Hypercellular areas (Antoni A type) and loose myxoid tissue (Antoni B type) coexist in tumor (Pushker et al. 2015).

9.1.2 Preferred Imaging Recommendations

1. CT: CT scanning should be used when the patients with eye symptoms are suspected to have retrobulbar lesions.
2. MRI: MR scanning should be done when the intraorbital mass is detected but not qualitatively diagnosed by CT scanning; MR scanning should be done when the relationship between intraorbital mass and adjacent structures is not clearly demonstrated by CT scanning.

D. Hao
Department of Radiology, The Affiliated Hospital of Qingdao University, Qingdao, China

Z. Wang (✉)
Department of Radiology, Beijing Friendship Hospital, Capital Medical University, Beijing, China
e-mail: cjr.wzhch@vip.163.com

Z. Zhang
Department of Radiology, Beijing Unicare ENT Hospital, Beijing, China

Z. Wang et al. (eds.), *Diagnostic Imaging of Ophthalmology*,
https://doi.org/10.1007/978-94-024-1060-0_9

9.1.3 Imaging Findings

1. CT findings: Schwannomas may arise in the intraconal or extraconal space. The majority features appear as oval, well defined, and the long axis oriented parallel to eye axis. The minority appearance is dumbbell-shape orbitocranial schwannomas involving the orbit and cavernous sinus simultaneously (Fig. 9.1). The appearances of schwannomas are nonspecific which mainly present as homogeneous isodense (Fig. 9.1a) and inhomogeneous enhanced on CT. The minority cases present as characteristic inhomogeneous masses with patches hypodense and inhomogeneous enhanced. The hypodense areas don't enhance. Very few schwannomas show cystic hypodense. There may be unenhanced or capsule enhanced.
2. MR findings: Schwannomas are seen as slightly hypointense (Figs. 9.1b and 9.2a) on T1WI, and slightly hyperintense on T2WI. The majority demonstrate heterogeneous signal (Figs. 9.1c and 9.2b) with patches hypointensity on T1WI

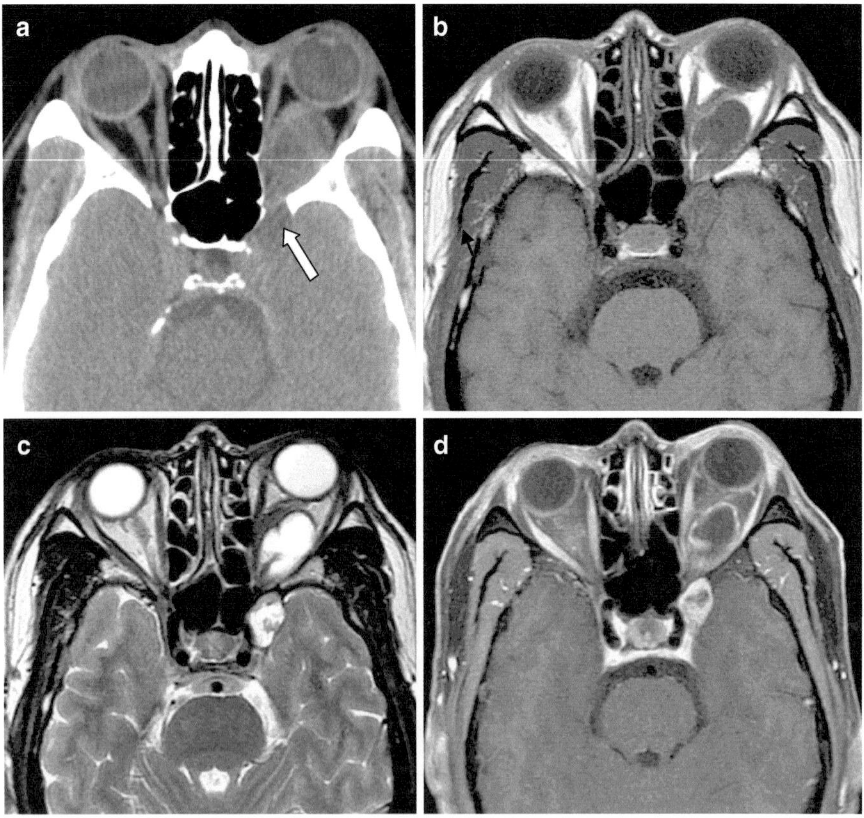

Fig. 9.1 Schwannoma in the left orbit. (**a**) Axial CT image in soft-tissue window shows an ovoid, well-demarcated homogeneous isodense mass in the left orbit. The left supraorbital fissure enlarges (*white arrow*). (**b**) Axial T1WI MR reveals a slightly hypointense and homogeneous mass. (**c**) Axial T2WI MR reveals a hyperintense mass, extending posteriorly to cavernous sinus. (**d**) Axial T1C+ MR shows heterogeneous intense signal enhancement of the mass

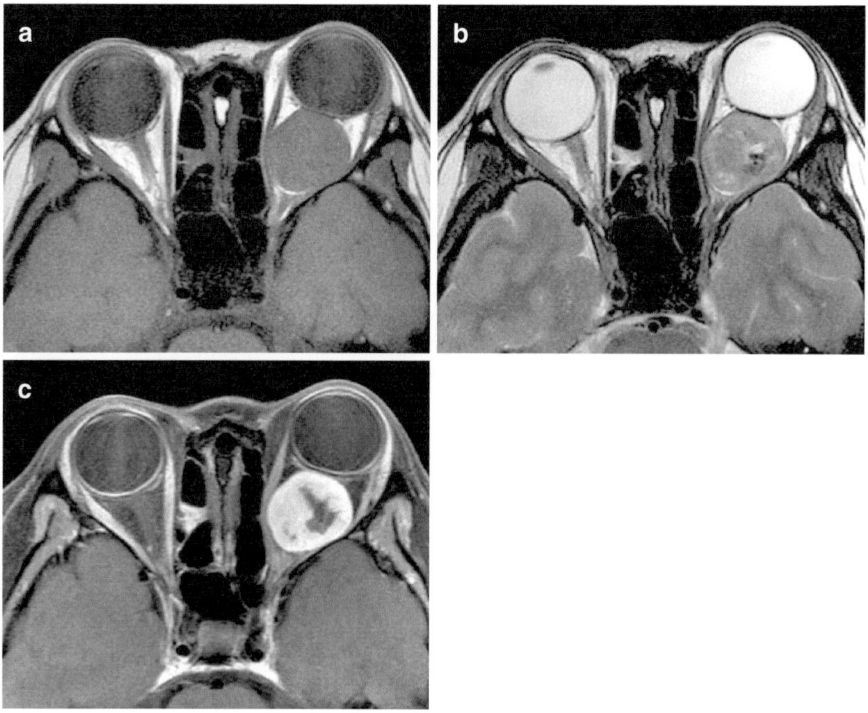

Fig. 9.2 Schwannoma in the left orbit. (**a**) Axial T1WI MR reveals an isointense and homogeneous mass in the left orbit. (**b**) Axial T2WI MR reveals heterogeneous moderate intensity of the mass. (**c**) Axial T1C+ MR with fat suppression shows heterogeneous enhancement of the mass. Patches of unenhanced area are seen in the mass

and hyperintensity on T2WI. The masses present inhomogeneous enhancement. The areas with slight hypointensity on T1WI show intense enhancement. The areas with hypointensity on T1WI don't enhance (Figs. 9.1d and 9.2c). Very few schwannomas show hypointensity on T1WI, hyperintensity on T2WI, and cystic unenhancement on T1 contrast examination (xian et al. 2010).

9.1.4 Diagnostic Checklist

CT can clearly demonstrate the location of the smaller schwannomas and their relationship with adjacent structure, but it is difficult to distinguish the bigger schwannomas from the adjacent structure with the similar density. CT is also difficult to differentiate the bigger schwannomas from other tumors in orbit.

MRI can demonstrate the signal of the schwannomas and their relationship with adjacent structure clearly, and it is easy to differentiate the schwannomas from other tumors. The qualitative diagnosis can be initially got from MR appearance.

9.2 Metastasis

9.2.1 Pathology

1. Unilateral or bilateral, but unilateral is more frequent.
2. The metastasis may originate from any site of the body. The most frequent primary tumors are lung, breast, digestive tract, and prostate carcinoma (Rajabi et al. 2015).

9.2.2 Preferred Imaging Recommendations

1. CT: CT scanning should be used when the patients with eye symptoms are suspected to have retrobulbar lesions.
2. MRI: Depending on the clinical history together with bony changes on CT, the qualitative diagnosis of orbital metastasis can be made. MR scanning should be further performed for delineating the extension of the lesion.

9.2.3 Imaging Findings

1. CT findings: Orbital metastasis mostly presents as a single soft-tissue mass in the orbital wall (Fig. 9.3a). The orbital wall may have osteogenic, osteolytic, or mixed bone destruction (Fig. 9.3b) with soft-tissue mass. The soft-tissue mass with necrosis may reveal heterogeneous density on CT imaging.
2. MR findings: Orbital metastasis demonstrates bone destruction and signal loss of the bone marrow. The lesion shows heterogeneous isointensity on T1WI (Fig. 9.3c) and heterogeneous hyperintensity on T2WI (Fig. 9.3d). If there are cystic necrosis areas, areas with hypointensity on T1WI and hyperintensity on T2WI may be seen. The lesion presents inhomogeneous enhancement. The cystic necrosis areas don't enhance.

9.2.4 Diagnostic Checklist

CT scanning demonstrates the bone destruction with soft-tissue mass in the orbital wall. The diagnosis can be clarified from CT combining with clinic history.

MR scanning should be further performed for delineating the tumor's extension. When metastasis is suspected, the additional specific examination should be performed to search for the primary tumor.

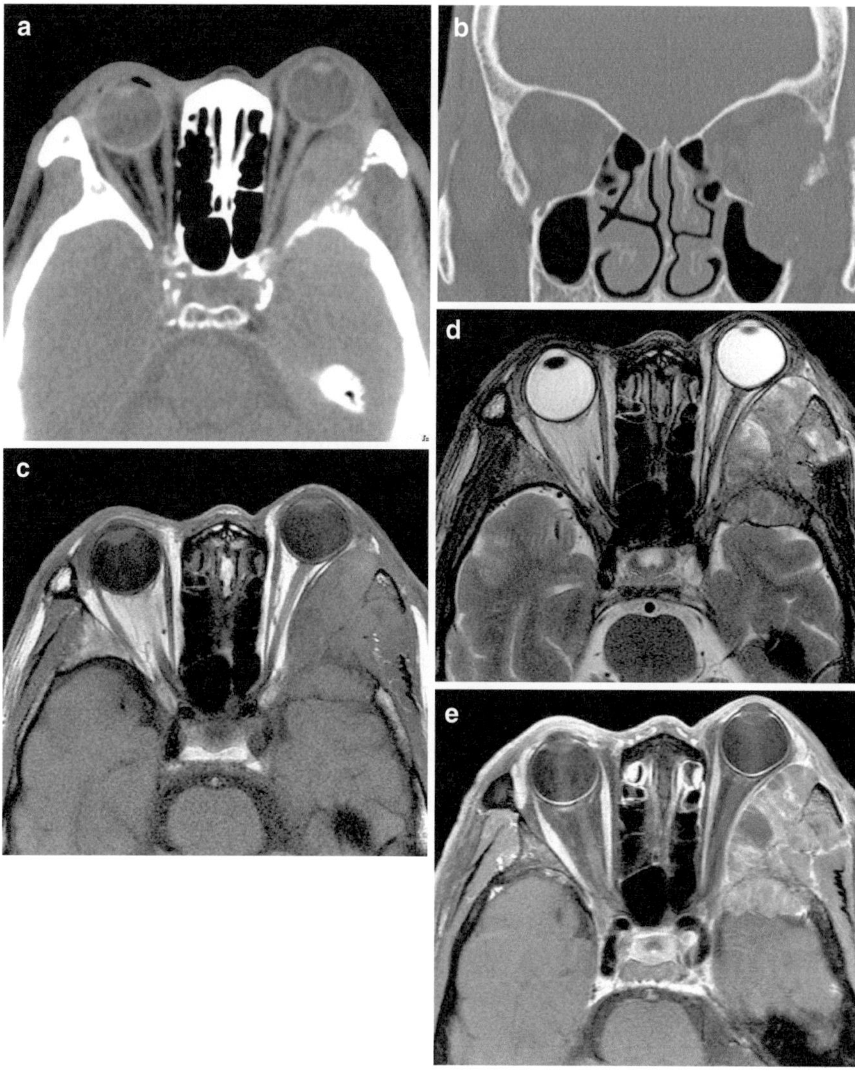

Fig. 9.3 Orbital metastasis. (**a**) Axial CT image in soft-tissue window demonstrates the osteolytic bone destruction with soft-tissue mass in the left greater wing of sphenoid bone. The mass is poor-demarcated and heterogeneous density. (**b**) Coronal CT image in bone window reveals the lesion involving the lateral and inferior orbital wall and the posterolateral wall of maxillary sinus. (**c**) Axial T1WI MR reveals a variably isointense to hypointense mass. The greater wing of sphenoid bone has bone destruction and signal loss of the bone marrow. (**d**) Axial T2WI MR reveals a variably isointense to hyperintense mass. (**e**) Axial T1C+ MR with fat suppression shows heterogeneous enhancement of the mass. The necrosis areas don't enhance. The tumor's extension is delineated clearly

9.3 Rhabdomyosarcoma

9.3.1 Pathology

1. Rhabdomyosarcoma is the primary orbital malignancy originating from mesoderm mesenchymal tissue.
2. Gross pathology shows fresh-red or slightly yellow mass with smooth surface and without connective tissue capsule.
3. Rhabdomyosarcomas are classified into three histologic types: embryonal, alveolar, and pleomorphic, with the embryonal accounting for 2/3.

9.3.2 Preferred Imaging Recommendations

1. CT: CT scanning should be used when the patients with rapidly progressing eye symptoms are suspected to have retrobulbar lesions.
2. MRI: When the intraorbital mass is detected by CT, MR scanning should be further performed for delineating the extension of the lesion.

9.3.3 Imaging Findings

1. CT findings: The tumor shows slight heterogeneous, poor-defined lobulated soft-tissue mass with adjacent osteolytic bone destruction (Fig. 9.4a, b). If there are cystic necrosis areas, hypodense patches may be seen.
2. MR findings: Orbital rhabdomyosarcomas demonstrate heterogeneous isointensity and hypointensity on T1WI (Fig. 9.4c) and heterogeneous hyperintensity on T2WI (Fig. 9.4d) with bone destruction. The lesions present moderate to marked enhancement. The patches of unenhanced cystic necrosis areas may present (Fig. 9.4e, f) (Mu et al. 2014).

9.3.4 Diagnostic Checklist

CT can clearly demonstrate the location and the adjacent bone erosion of the rhabdomyosarcoma. The boundary of the tumor is unclear for the similar density with adjacent soft tissue.

MR can reveal the signal characteristics of the tumor and the relationship with adjacent structures. The qualitative diagnosis can be initially got from tightly combing the clinical profile with CT and MR imaging.

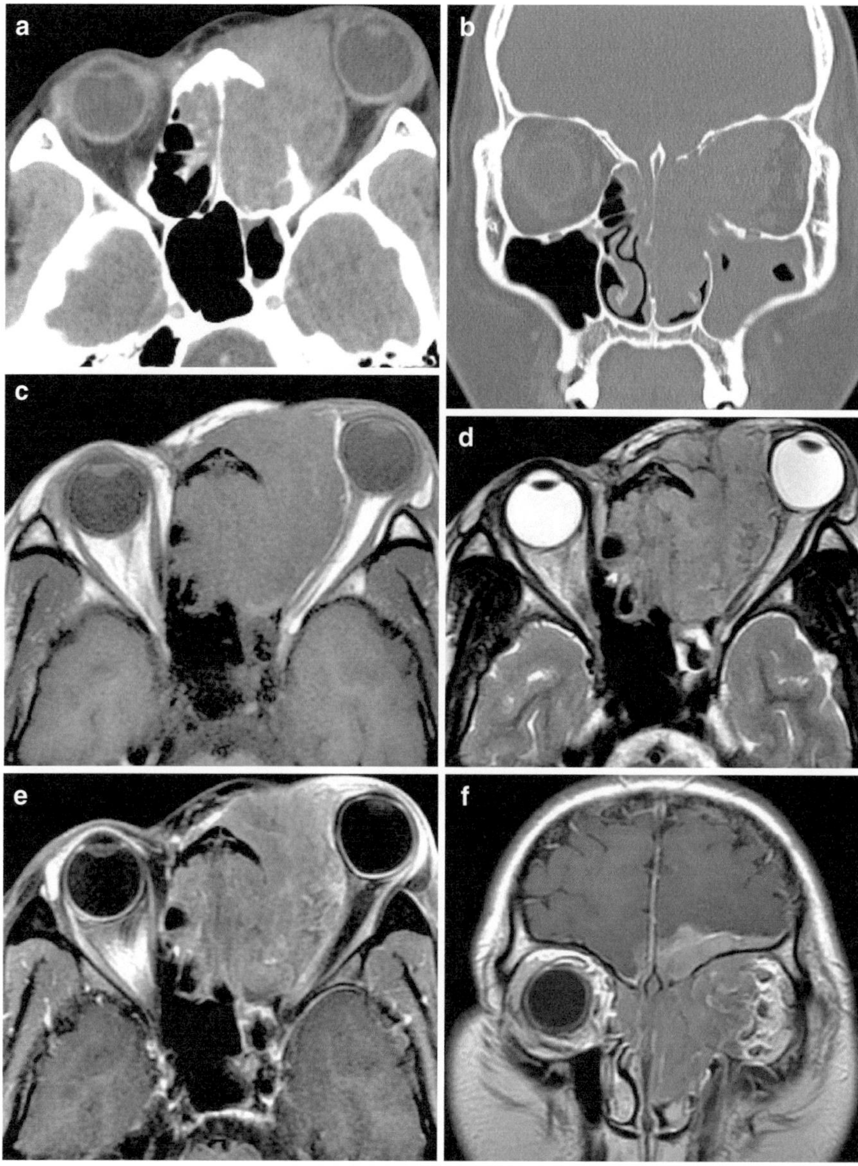

Fig. 9.4 Orbital rhabdomyosarcoma. (**a**) Axial CT image in soft-tissue window reveals large irregular soft-tissue mass in the left orbit. The mass is poor-demarcated and heterogeneous density. The tumor extends into the left ethmoid sinus. (**b**) Coronal CT image in bone window reveals bone destruction in the medial orbital wall. The lesion extends into the ethmoid sinuses and the nasal cavities. The lesion has indistinct margins with intraorbital structures. (**c**) Axial T1WI MR reveals a heterogeneous isointense mass in the left orbit. The intraorbital structures are compressed. (**d**) Axial T2WI MR reveals a heterogeneous hyperintense mass. (**e**) Axial T1C+ MR with fat suppression shows heterogeneous moderate enhancement of the mass. The tumor is poor-demarcated. (**f**) Coronal T1C+ MR reveals parameningeal rhabdomyosarcoma widely extending into the orbit and nasal cavities

9.4 Chloroma

9.4.1 Pathology

1. Chloroma is also called granulocytic sarcoma, which is a special kind of acute myelogenous leukemia.
2. The disease is called chloroma because the myeloperoxidase with the tumor imparts a green hue to it after exposure to air.
3. Chloroma can arise at any part of the body. The skull base and orbit are frequently involved.
4. The type M5 is the common subgroup of extramedullary infiltration of acute myelogenous leukemia (Ke et al. 2011).

9.4.2 Preferred Imaging Recommendations

1. CT: CT scanning should be used when the patients with relative eye symptoms are suspected to have retrobulbar lesions.
2. MRI: When the lesion is detected by CT, MR scanning should be further performed for delineating the extension of the lesion and the relationship with adjacent structure.

9.4.3 Imaging Findings

1. CT findings: Orbital chloromas typically involve extraconal space (Fig. 9.5a) and can present as single or multiple masses involving the craniofacial bones (Fig. 9.5b), with osteolytic bone destruction or bone remodeling. Radial bone spicule is seldom seen (Fig. 9.5c).
2. MR findings: Orbital chloromas demonstrate homogeneous isointensity on T1WI (Fig. 9.5d, f) and slight hyperintensity on T2WI (Fig. 9.5e, g). The signal loss of bone marrow may be seen on the greater wing of sphenoid bone, petrous apex, zygoma, and clivus (Fig. 9.5d, f), which highly indicates chloroma. The lesions present moderate enhancement.

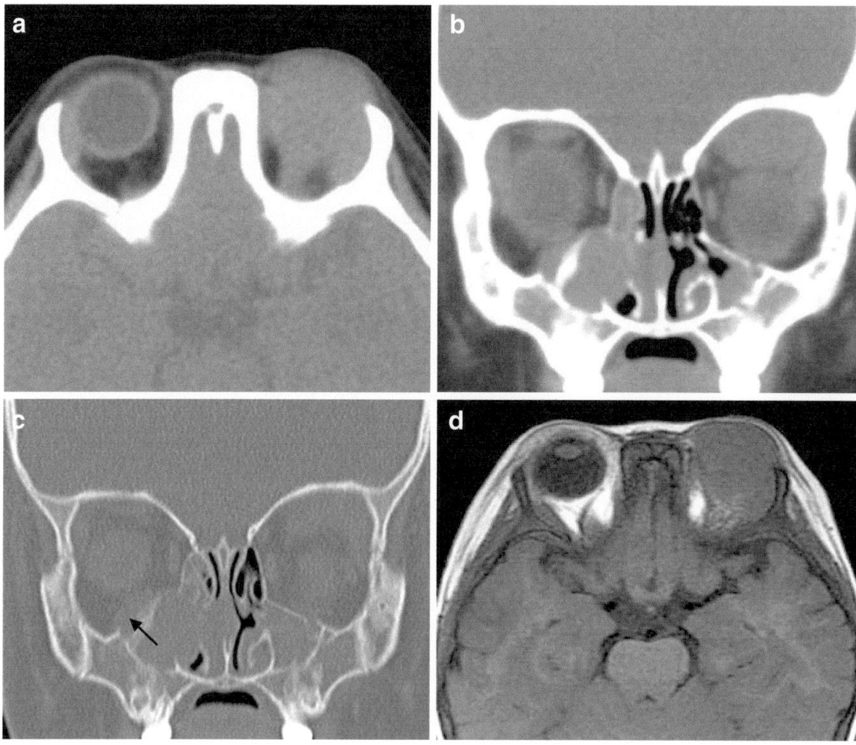

Fig. 9.5 Orbital chloroma. (**a**) Axial CT image in soft-tissue window reveals homogeneous soft-tissue density mass in the left orbit. (**b**) Coronal CT image in soft-tissue window reveals multiple lesions involving the left orbit and bilateral maxillary sinuses. (**c**) Coronal CT image in bone window reveals slightly rough margin and osteolytic bone destruction (*black arrow*) in the involved bone. (**d**) Axial T1WI MR reveals a homogenous isointense mass in the left orbit. The bilateral greater wings of sphenoid bone demonstrate bone marrow signal loss. (**e**) Axial T2WI MR reveals a homogeneous slight hyperintense mass. (**f**) Axial T1WI MR reveals isointense lesion in the bilateral maxillary sinuses. The clivus demonstrates bone marrow signal loss (*white arrow*). (**g**) Axial T2WI MR reveals slightly hyperintense lesions in the bilateral maxillary sinuses

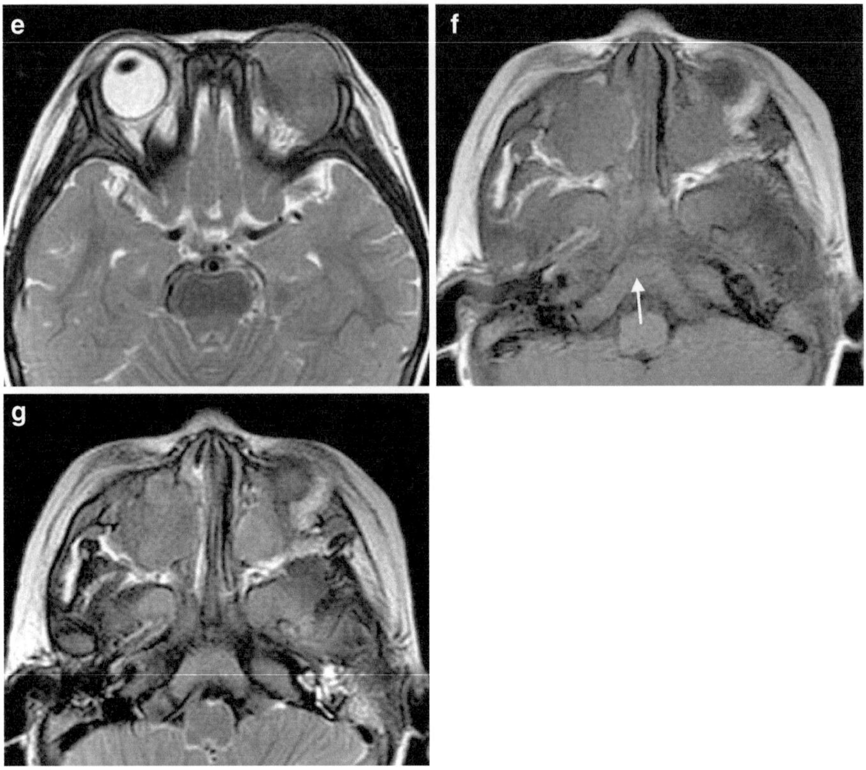

Fig. 9.5 (continued)

9.4.4 Diagnostic Checklist

CT can clearly demonstrate the location and the adjacent bone erosion of the chloroma. It is difficult to differentiate chloroma from other orbital tumors sometimes.

MR can reveal the signal characteristics and the relationship with adjacent structure of the tumor. The signal change of bone marrow in skull base can also be seen on MR. MR can improve the diagnostic accuracy of this disease.

The chloroma can occur several months before the positive blood test of leukemia. The chloroma should be considered for children with orbital tumor, even if the peripheral blood test is normal.

9.5 Pleomorphic Adenoma of the Lacrimal Gland

9.5.1 Pathology

1. Majority originate in the orbit lobe of the lacrimal gland. Minority originate in the palpebral lobe of the lacrimal gland or the ectopic lacrimal gland.
2. Majority are lobulated masses with capsule and nodular bosselated. Myxoid and fibrous tissue coexist in tumor on pathological section.
3. Diverse components include mesodermal epithelial and exoderm mesenchymal.

9.5.2 Preferred Imaging Recommendations

1. CT: CT scanning should be used when the patients with relative eye symptoms are suspected to have lacrimal fossa lesions.
2. MRI: When the lacrimal mass is detected by CT, MR scanning should be further performed for clarifying the qualitative diagnosis and origin and delineating the extension of the lesion.

9.5.3 Imaging Findings

1. CT findings: The tumor shows a homogeneous-density soft-tissue mass in the lacrimal fossa (Figs. 9.6a, and 9.7a). The mass is regular-shaped, round or oval, and circumscribed with scalloped remodeling of the bony lacrimal fossa (Figs. 9.6b, and 9.7b) (Gibson et al. 2007).
2. MR findings: The tumor demonstrates isointensity on T1WI (Figs. 9.6c, d and 9.7c) and isointensity or hyperintensity on T2WI with hypointense capsule (Figs. 9.6e, and 9.7d) and cystic areas. The tumor presents moderate to marked enhancement (Figs. 9.6f, and 9.7e, f).

9.5.4 Diagnostic Checklist

CT can demonstrate the location, shape, and adjacent bone remodeling of the tumor and help for qualitative diagnosis. It is difficult to differentiate pleomorphic adenoma from schwannoma sometimes.

MR can reveal the signal characteristics of the tumor and the relationship with adjacent structures. CT combining with MR can improve the diagnostic accuracy of this disease.

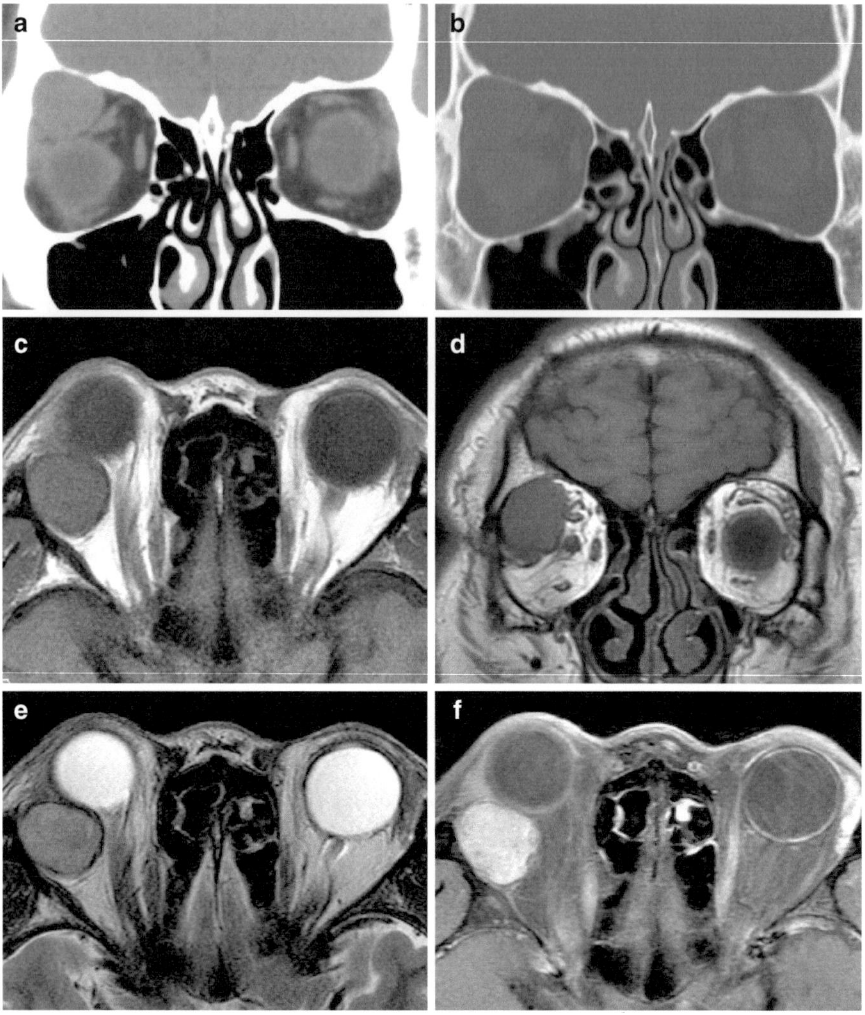

Fig. 9.6 Pleomorphic adenoma of the right lacrimal gland. (**a**) Coronal CT image in soft-tissue window reveals a round, well-defined homogeneous soft-tissue density mass in the right lacrimal fossa. (**b**) Coronal CT image in bone window reveals the tumor with smooth margin and scalloped remodeling of the bony lacrimal fossa. (**c**) Axial T1WI MR reveals a homogenous isointense mass. (**d**) Coronal T1WI MR reveals the mass in the lacrimal fossa that compresses the adjacent structures. (**e**) Axial T2WI MR reveals a homogeneous hyperintense mass with hypointense capsule. (**f**) Axial T1C+ MR with fat suppression shows homogeneous marked enhancement of the mass

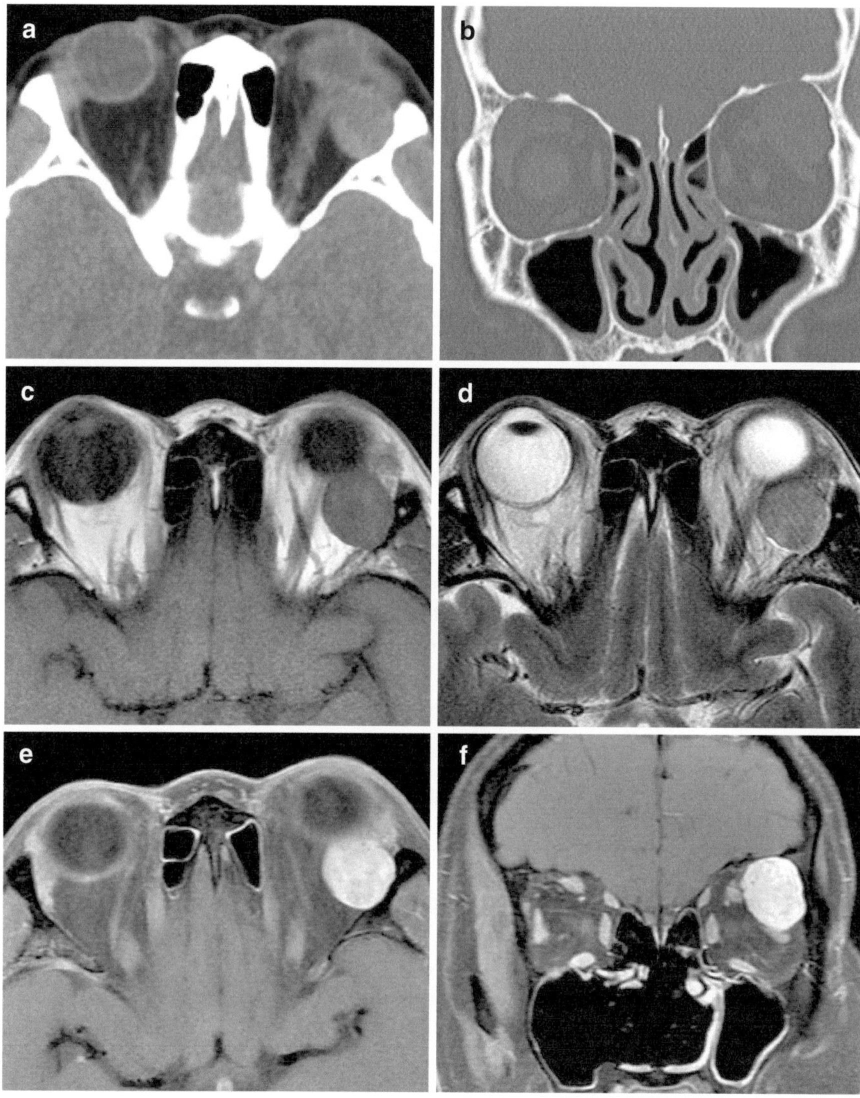

Fig. 9.7 Pleomorphic adenoma of the left lacrimal gland. (**a**) Axial CT image in soft-tissue window reveals a well-defined homogeneous soft-tissue density mass in the left lacrimal fossa. (**b**) Coronal CT image in bone window reveals the tumor with smooth margin and scalloped remodeling of the bony lacrimal fossa. (**c**) Axial T1WI MR reveals a homogenous isointense mass. (**d**) Axial T2WI MR reveals a well-defined and slightly hyperintense mass with hypointense capsule at the front and medial margins. (**e**) Axial T1C+ MR with fat suppression shows marked enhancement of the mass. (**f**) Coronal T1C+ MR with fat suppression shows homogeneous marked enhancement of the mass

9.6 Adenoid Cystic Carcinoma of the Lacrimal Gland

9.6.1 Pathology

1. Adenoid cystic carcinoma is the most common lacrimal gland malignant epithelial tumor which originates in the exoderm epithelial.
2. Adenoid cystic carcinoma is a tumor without capsule. Papillary and cystic structures coexist in tumor on pathological section.
3. Adenoid cystic carcinoma often infiltrates adjacent structures through vessels and nerves. Adenoid cystic carcinoma has a strong propensity for spreading to intracranal, temporal fossa and paranasal sinuses.

9.6.2 Preferred Imaging Recommendations

1. CT: CT scanning should be used when the patients with relative eye symptoms are suspected to have lacrimal fossa lesions.
2. MRI: When the lacrimal mass is detected by CT, MR scanning should be further performed for delineating the extension of the lesion.

9.6.3 Imaging Findings

1. CT findings: The majority appear as irregular masses. The minority appear as ovoid or round, poor-demarcated masses with bone erosion, or saw-tooth destructive bone destruction in adjacent orbital walls (Figs. 9.8 and 9.9a, b). The masses often grow towards orbit apex along the orbital wall. Sometimes the tumors spread intracranially.
2. MR findings: The tumor demonstrates heterogeneous isointensity on T1WI (Figs. 9.9c and 9.10a) and isointensity to slight hyperintensity on T2WI (Figs. 9.9d and 9.10b). The tumor presents heterogeneous moderate to marked enhancement (Figs. 9.9e, f and 9.10c). When the tumor spreads intracranially, various enhancement of meningeal or brain parenchyma can be seen (Wang et al. 2013).

9.6.4 Diagnostic Checklist

CT can demonstrate the location, shape, and adjacent bone destruction of the tumor and help for diagnosis.

MR can reveal the signal characteristics of the tumor and the relationship with adjacent structures. CT combining with MR can improve the diagnostic accuracy of this disease.

9.7 Sphenoid Ridge Meningioma

9.7.1 Pathology

1. Sphenoid ridge meningioma is also called a plaque meningioma, which mostly originates from orbital periosteum.
2. The tumor shows purple-red with rich blood supply and local dural hypervascularity sometimes.
3. The most common type is epithelial type. The tumor can invade adjacent bone, fat, and muscle (Russell and Benjamin 2008).

9.7.2 Preferred Imaging Recommendations

1. CT: CT scanning should be used when the patients with relative eye symptoms are suspected to have retrobulbar lesions.
2. MRI: When the lesion is detected by CT, MR scanning should be further performed for delineating the extension of the lesion.

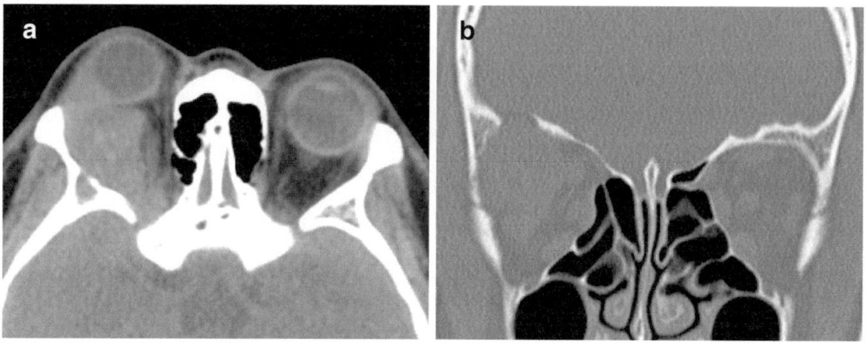

Fig. 9.8 Adenoid cystic carcinoma of the right lacrimal gland. (**a**) Axial CT image in soft-tissue window reveals a poor-defined, irregular soft-tissue density mass in the right lacrimal fossa. (**b**) Coronal CT image in bone window reveals bone destruction in adjacent superior and lateral orbital walls

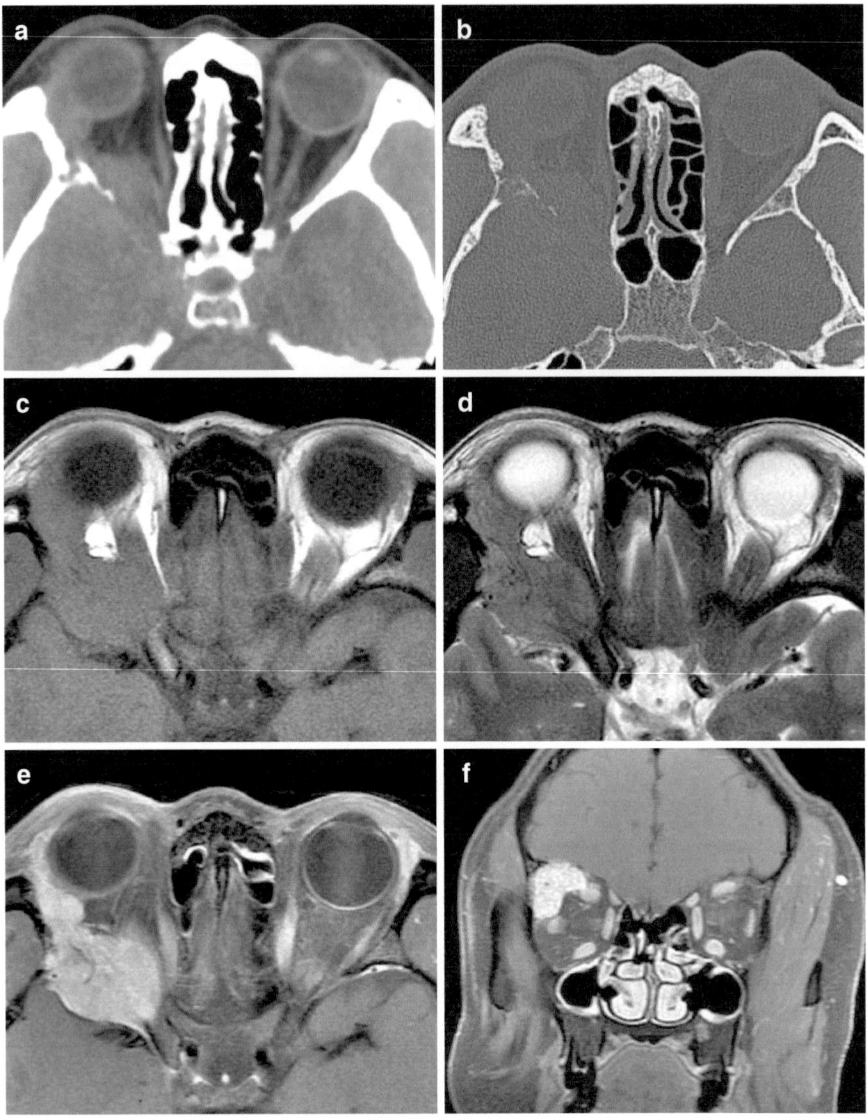

Fig. 9.9 Adenoid cystic carcinoma of the right lacrimal gland. (**a**). Axial CT image in soft-tissue window reveals a poor-defined, irregular soft-tissue density mass in the right lacrimal fossa. (**b**) Axial CT image in bone window reveals the tumor with rough margin and bone destruction in adjacent lateral orbital wall. (**c**) Axial T1WI MR reveals a homogenous isointense mass with bone destruction in adjacent lateral orbital wall. (**d**) Axial T2WI MR reveals an isointense and slightly hyperintense mass with extension to orbit apex. (**e**) Axial T1C+ MRI with fat saturation shows the tumor marked enhanced. (**f**) Coronal T1C+ MR with fat suppression shows heterogeneous intense signal enhancement of the mass in the lacrimal fossa

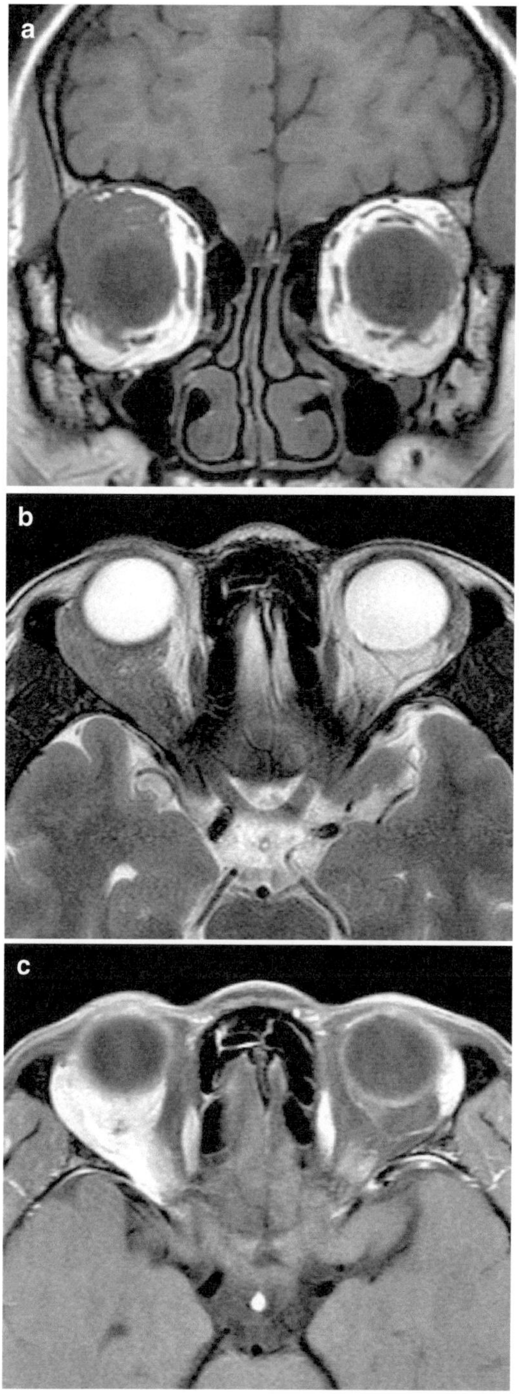

Fig. 9.10 Adenoid cystic carcinoma of the right lacrimal gland. (**a**) Coronal T1WI MR reveals an inhomogeneous isointense mass in the super-lateral quadrant of the right orbit. (**b**) Axial T2WI MR reveals an inhomogeneous isointense mass partially surrounding the right eyeball. (**c**) Axial T1C+ MR with fat suppression shows heterogeneous marked enhancement of the mass

9.7.3 Imaging Findings

1. CT findings: Sphenoid ridge meningioma appears as a sheetlike, poor-demarcated soft-tissue density mass with adjacent hyperostosis around the greater wing of sphenoid bone (Figs. 9.11 and 9.12a, b).
2. MR findings: The mass mostly demonstrates isointensity on T1WI (Figs. 9.11c and 9.12c) and isointensity and hypointensity on T2WI (Figs. 9.11d and 9.12d). Bone marrow signal loss and hyperostosis are seen in the greater wing of sphenoid bone and the involved bone. The tumor presents marked enhancement with intracranial "dural-tail" (Figs. 9.11e, f and 9.12e, f).

9.7.4 Diagnostic Checklist

CT can demonstrate the shape and extension of sphenoid ridge meningioma. The bone change is characteristic and can help for qualitatively diagnosis.

MR can demonstrate intracranial changes and clarify the extension of the tumor.

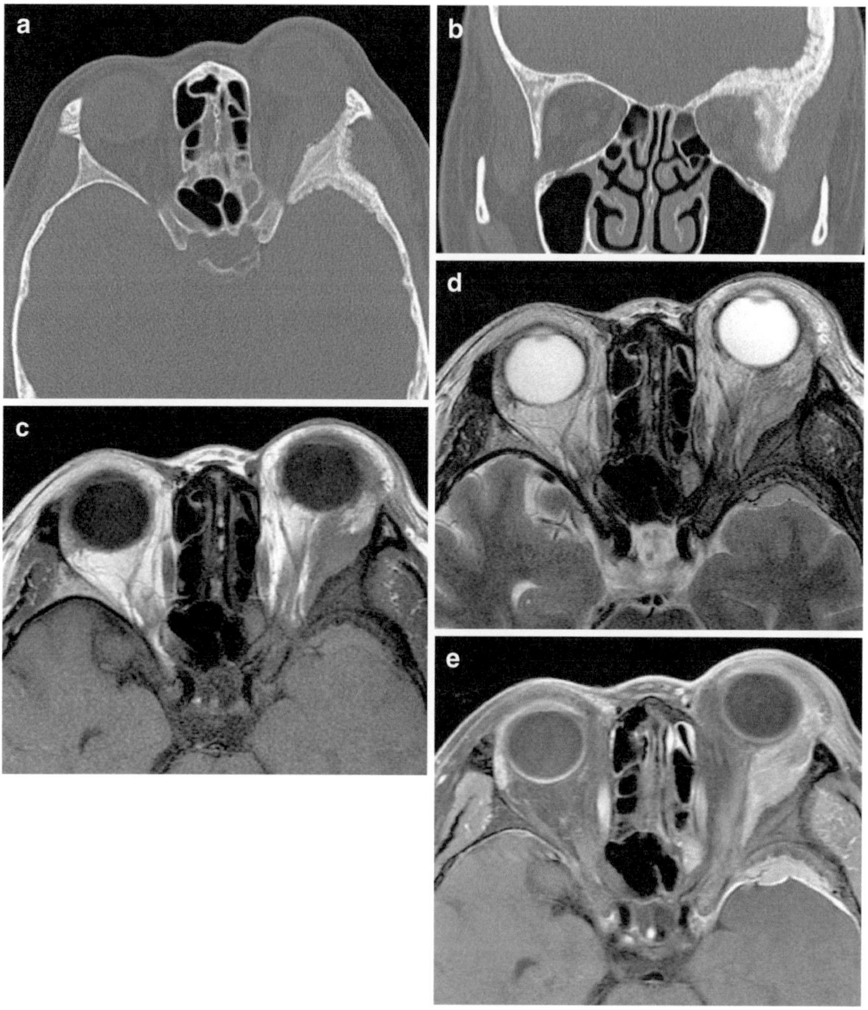

Fig. 9.11 Left sphenoid ridge meningioma. (**a**) Axial CT image in bone window reveals hyperostosis in left greater wing of sphenoid bone with rough margin. (**b**) Coronal CT image in bone window reveals hyperostosis in left greater wing of sphenoid bone, superior orbital wall, and partial frontal bone with rough margin. (**c**) Axial T1WI MR reveals an isointense sheetlike mass around left greater wing of sphenoid bone. Bone marrow signal loss is seen in the left greater wing of sphenoid bone. (**d**) Axial T2WI MR reveals a slight hyperintense mass. (**e**) Axial T1C+ MR with fat suppression shows marked enhancement of the mass with the thick enhanced left temporal pole meningeal and "dural-tail"

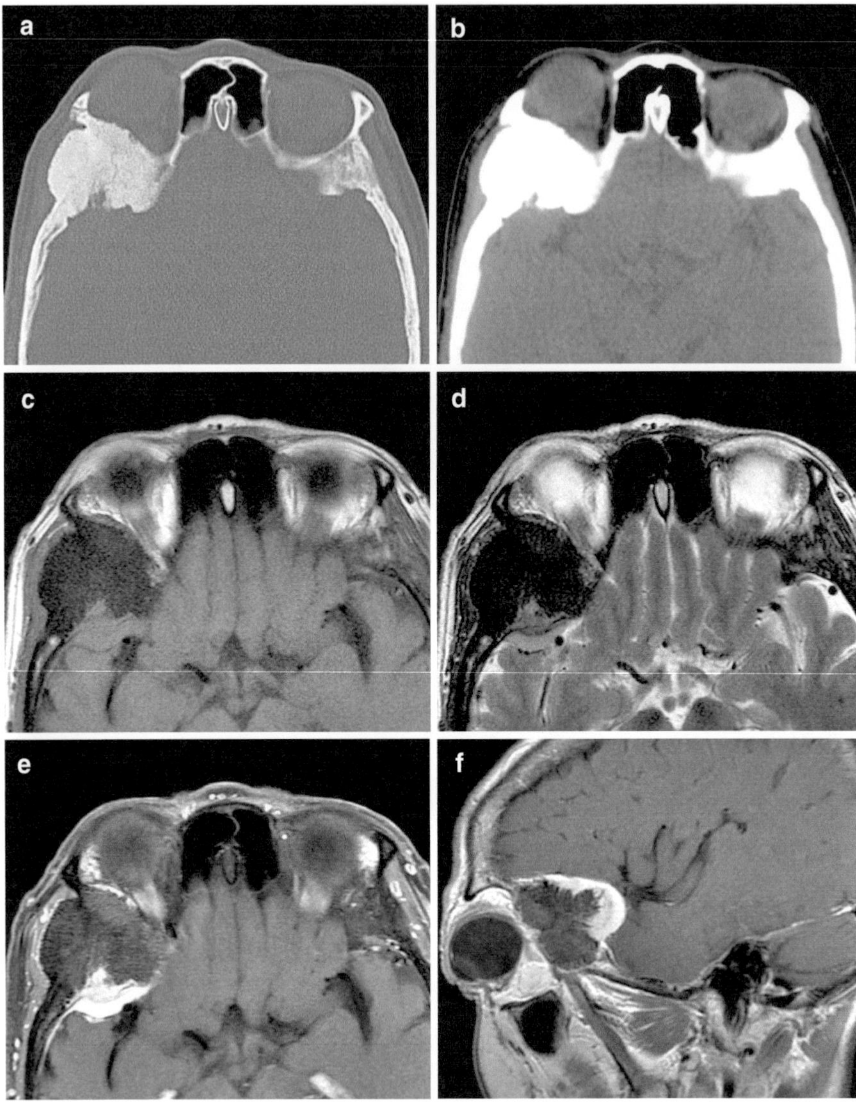

Fig. 9.12 Right sphenoid ridge meningioma. (**a**) Axial CT image in bone window reveals hyperostosis in right greater wing of sphenoid bone. (**b**) Coronal CT image in soft-tissue window reveals a few soft-tissue density around right greater wing of sphenoid bone. (**c**) Axial T1WI MR reveals round hypointensity of the right greater wing of sphenoid bone surrounded by strip isointensity. (**d**) Axial T2WI MR reveals hypointense greater wing of sphenoid bone surrounded by isointense soft-tissue mass. (**e**) Axial T1C+ MR with fat suppression shows sheetlike marked enhancement around the right greater wing of sphenoid bone with "dural-tail." (**f**) Sagittal T1C+ MR shows marked enhancement of the soft-tissue mass around the right greater wing of sphenoid bone

9.8 Osteoma of the Orbital Wall

9.8.1 Pathology

1. Gross pathology demonstrates osteoma as a rocklike hard mass projecting into orbit and paranasal sinus cavity.
2. Microscopic features of the osteoma include three types: ivory-type osteoma, which is composed of mature bone; cancellous-type osteoma, which is composed of marginal dense bone and central radial bone marrow; and mix-type osteoma, which is composed of bone and fibrous tissues.

9.8.2 Preferred Imaging Recommendations

1. CT: CT scanning is the first choice for demonstrating osteoma, because it has obvious advantage for diagnosing bone-forming lesions.
2. MRI: When the osteoma is large, MR scanning should be performed to demonstrate intracranial and other important structures.

9.8.3 Imaging Findings

CT findings: The osteoma demonstrates intraorbital heterogeneous bone density mass with sharp margin and corresponding orbital wall deformity. The mass mostly involves the ipsilateral nasal cavity and paranasal cavity and compresses the intraorbital structures (Fig. 9.13).

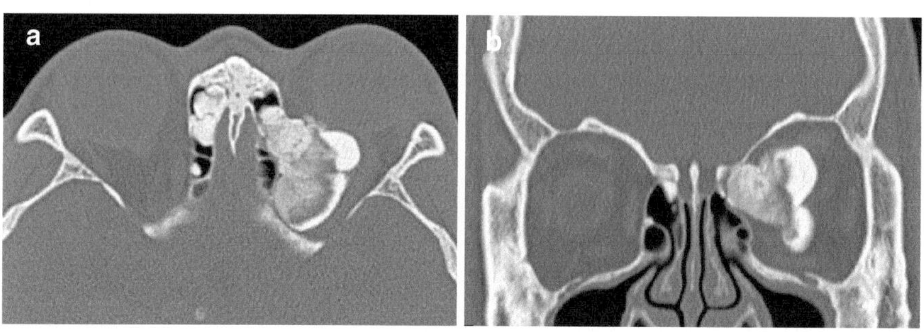

Fig. 9.13 Osteoma of the orbital wall. (**a**) Axial CT image in bone window reveals an irregular heterogeneous bone density mass in the left orbit. A lump of bone density mass is also seen in the right ethmoid sinus. (**b**) Coronal CT image in bone window reveals the left mass compressing the medial wall of the orbit and protruding into the orbit cavity

9.8.4 Diagnostic Checklist

CT can demonstrate the size, location, shape, and adjacent bone destruction of the tumor and help for differentiating the osteoma from other intraorbital tumors.

When the osteoma is large, MR scanning should be performed to demonstrate intracranial structures, but MR scanning is not a routine method.

References

Gibson A, Mavrikakis I, Rootman J, et al. Lacrimal gland pleomorphic adenomas with low-density zones resembling cystic change on computed tomography. Ophthal Plast Reconstr Surg. 2007;23(3):234–5.

Ke YF, Zhang H, Song GX. Clinical analysis of orbital chloroma. Chinese J Ophthalmol. 2011;47(9):811–4.

Mu XT, Wang H, Li YY, et al. Magnetic resonance imaging and DWI features of orbital rhabdomyosarcoma. Eye Sci. 2014;29(1):6–11.

Pushker N, Khurana S, Kashyap S, et al. Orbital schwannoma: a clinicopathologic study. Int Ophthalmol. 2015;35(4):481–6.

Rajabi MT, Saeedi-Anari G, Ramezani F, et al. Orbital metastatic osteosarcoma. Arch Iran Med. 2015;18(2):123–6.

Russell SM, Benjamin V. Medial sphenoid ridge meningiomas: classification, microsurgical anatomy, operative nuances, and long-term surgical outcome in 35 consecutive patients. Neurosurgery. 2008;62(3 Suppl 1):38–50.

Wang F, Sun FY, Guo XX, et al. Imaging feature and clinical histological analysis of 12 adenoid cystic carcinoma of the lacrimal gland. Chinese J Ophthalmol. 2013;49(1):47–51.

Xian J, Zhang Z, Wang Z, et al. Evaluation of MR imaging findings differentiating cavernous haemangiomas from schwannomas in the orbit. Eur Radiol. 2010;20(9):2221–8.

Chapter 10
Neuro-Ophthalmology

Yiqun Zhan, Fengyuan Man, Jing Feng, and Zhengyu Zhang

10.1 Optic Neuritis

10.1.1 Pathological Characteristics

1. Including multiple sclerosis with optic neuritis, nonspecific solidary optic neuritis, etc. The exact cause of optic neuritis is unknown. However, optic neuritis is generally believed to be an autoimmune disorder.
2. Papilledema can be found in the acute stage. Optic atrophy follows if there is repeated attack and protracted course of the disease.
3. Acute features include demyelination, axonal injury, cholesterol crystal, and infiltration with macrophages, lymphocytes, as well as plasma cells. Chronic features include optic atrophy, gliosis and scar, and even the formation of necrosis cavum (Shams and Plant 2009).

Y. Zhan
Department of Neurovascular Surgery, The PLA Rocket Force General Hospital, Beijing, China

F. Man (✉)
Department of Medical Imaging, The PLA Rocket Force General Hospital, Beijing, China
e-mail: manfengyuan@yeah.net

J. Feng
Department of Ophthalmology, The PLA Rocket Force General Hospital, Beijing, China

Z. Zhang
Department of Radiology, Beijing Unicare ENT Hospital, Beijing, China

Z. Wang et al. (eds.), *Diagnostic Imaging of Ophthalmology*,
https://doi.org/10.1007/978-94-024-1060-0_10

10.1.2 The Choice of Imaging Modality

1. MRI: For patients with acute vision decline, unenhanced MRI scan is suggested first, while in the acute stage enhanced MRI is used.
2. CT scanning has a very limited role.

10.1.3 Imaging Findings

MRI findings: Unilateral diffuse minimally expanded or nonexpanded optic nerve can be seen in over 70% of images, mostly involving the middle intraorbital segment (Fig. 10.1a), with segmental hyperintensities most prominent on T2WI image (Fig. 10.1b). The lesion can be enhanced in the postgadolinium image (Fig. 10.1c). In a few cases the optic nerve sheath can be enhanced presenting a "double-track sign." The optic neuritis often can be the initial episode of multiple sclerosis and optical neuromyelitis, so intracranial and intraspinal exams should be done at the same time.

10.1.4 Comments

If young and middle-aged patients present with acute vision decline and MRI shows segmental hyperintensities in the optic nerve, enhanced obviously postgadolinium, then optic neuritis is indicated. Meanwhile, intracranial and intraspinal exams should be done to see if multiple sclerosis or optical neuromyelitis is suggested.

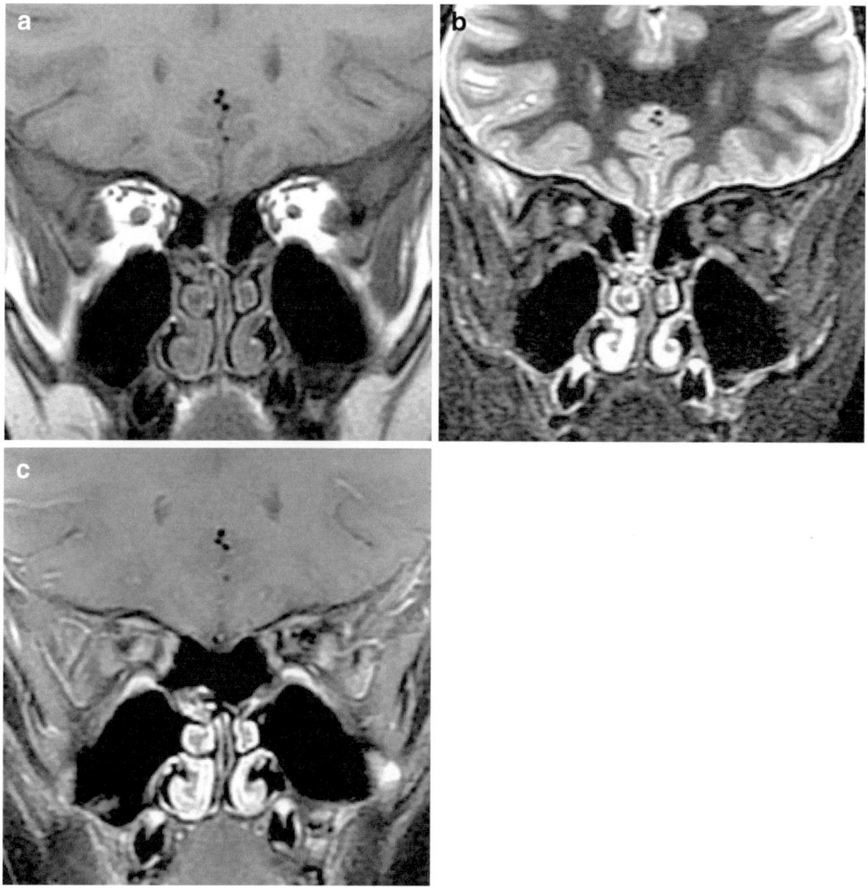

Fig. 10.1 Right optic neuritis. (**a**) Coronal T1-weighted image demonstrates the *right* optic nerve expansion compared to the *left*. (**b**) Coronal, short time inversion recovery (STIR) image demonstrates increased signal in the right optic nerve. (**c**) Coronal, fat-suppressed, postcontrast MRI image demonstrates significant enhancement in the right optic nerve, with mildly coarse margin

10.2 Optic Nerve Glioma

10.2.1 Pathological Characteristics

1. Optic nerve glioma, originating from the glial cells in the optic nerve, is a kind of benign or low-grade malignant tumor.
2. According to the age of onset, optic nerve glioma can be classified into two categories: the childhood optic nerve glioma and the adult optic nerve glioma. The former is more common and is mostly pilocytic astrocytoma. The adult form is very rare and usually aggressive.
3. The section of the lesions often appears white. The optic nerve is enlarged, surrounded by arachnoid tissues with different thicknesses, which are covered with tight dura mater.

10.2.2 The Choice of Imaging Modality

1. CT: If the patient presents related ocular symptoms and clinical examination shows retrobulbar disease, CT is often the first investigation performed.
2. MRI: Once the CT scan reveals a mass image in the optic nerve area, MRI can be further performed to clarify the nature of the lesions, involving the origin and scope.

10.2.3 Imaging Findings

1. CT findings: CT scan usually reveals a soft-tissue mass in the optic nerve area, with homogeneous density, consistent with the long axis of the optic nerves (Fig. 10.2a, b). If the medial segment of the optic canal is involved, then optic canal enlargement can be seen.
2. MRI findings: On T1-weighted images, optic nerve gliomas are usually homogeneous hypointense (Figs. 10.2c and 10.3a), and on T2-weighted images homogeneous hyperintense (Figs. 10.2d and 10.3b). Sometimes the subarachnoid space around the optic nerve can be seen widened and expanded because of tumor compression, and the lesions are enhanced to varying degrees, from non-enhanced to significantly enhanced (Figs. 10.2e and 10.3c, d). The optic canal-involved and intracranial lesions may demonstrate a dumbbell-like appearance (Walrath et al. 2008).

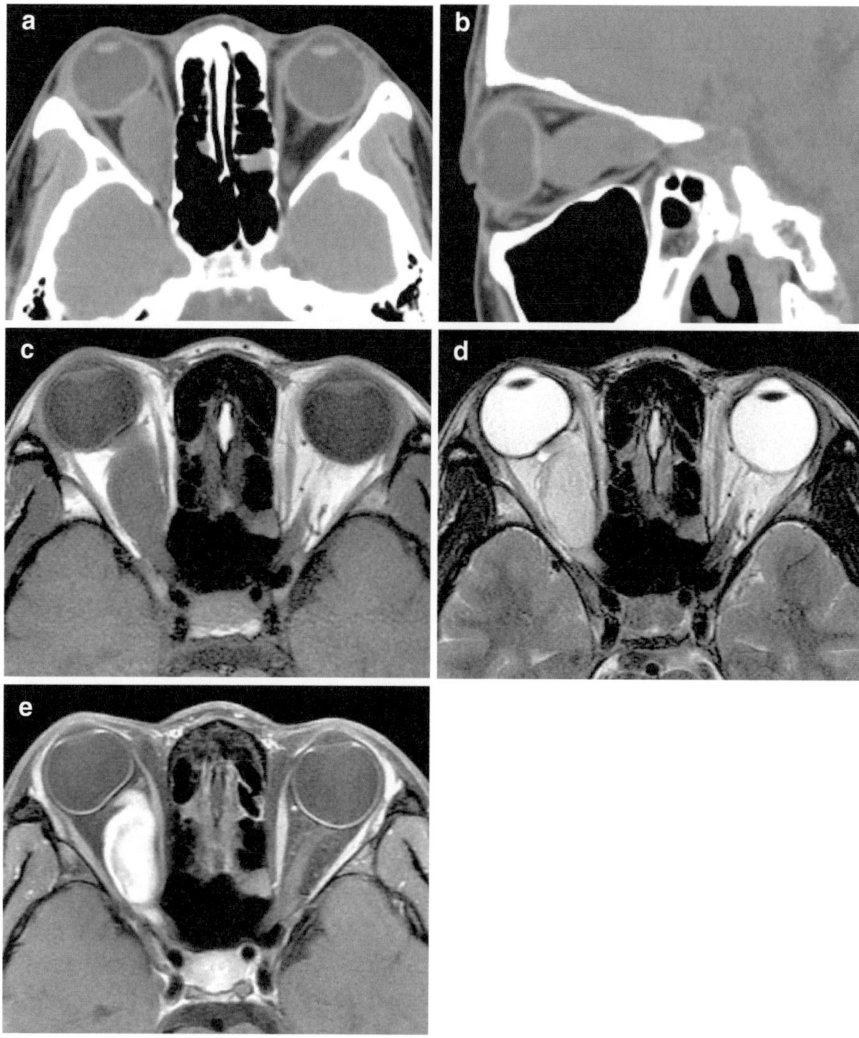

Fig. 10.2 Optic nerve glioma. (**a**) Cross-sectional CT soft-tissue window shows that the lesion in the right orbit, along the optic nerve, appears isodense. (**b**) Oblique sagittal CT soft-tissue window shows that the lesion is along the optic nerve and rodlike. (**c**) Cross-sectional T1-weighted MRI shows that the lesion in the right orbit is relatively homogeneous hypointense, pressing the back part of the eyeball. (**d**) Cross-sectional T2-weighted MRI shows that the lesion is homogeneous hyperintense. (**e**) Cross-sectional, fat-suppressed, postcontrast MRI image reveals intense homogeneous enhancement of the lesion

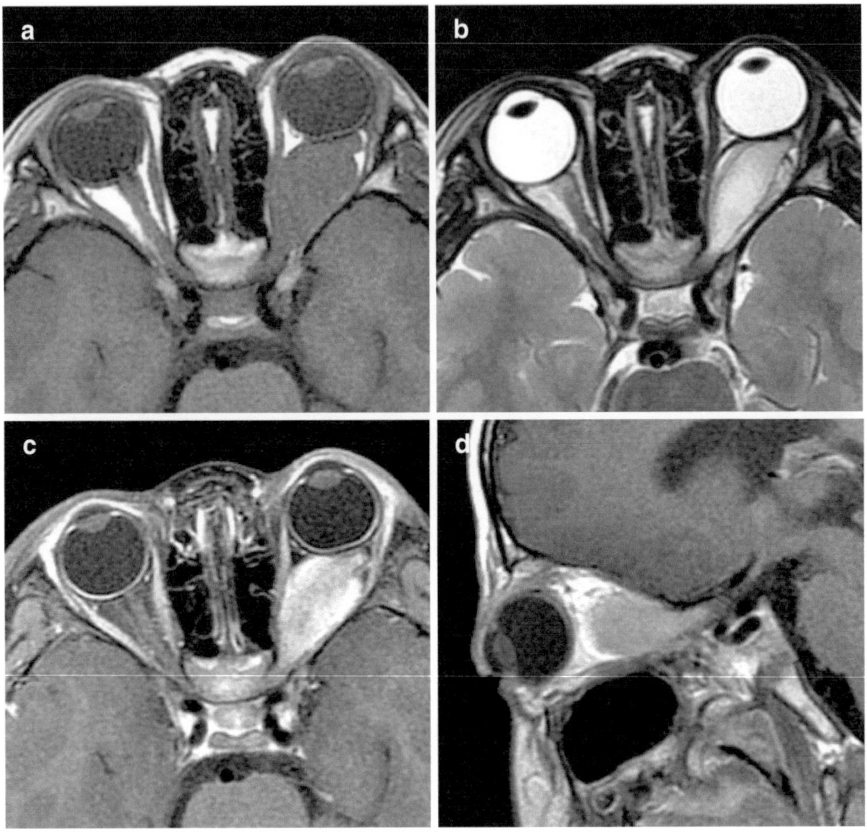

Fig. 10.3 Optic nerve glioma. (**a**) Cross-sectional T1-weighted MRI reveals an isointense mass along the optic nerve area. (**b**) Cross-sectional T2-weighted MRI shows a hyperintense lesion. (**c**) Cross-sectional, fat-suppressed, postcontrast MRI image reveals a lesion significantly enhanced. (**d**) Oblique sagittal, postcontrast MRI images demonstrate that the lesion grows along the optic nerve

10.2.4 Comments

The diagnosis of optic nerve glioma should be considered in any patient presenting with relevant symptoms when CT shows a mass along the optic nerve area. MRI is further performed to assess the range of the lesion and to help confirm the diagnosis.

10.3 Optic Nerve Sheath Meningioma (ONSM)

10.3.1 *Pathological Characteristics*

1. ONSMs arise from the optic nerve arachnoid fibroblasts or endothelial cells on the inside of the dura. It is mostly benign, and few can be malignant.
2. ONSMs appear light red, with no capsule. The tumor typically has a smooth contour.

10.3.2 *The Choice of Imaging Modality*

1. CT: If the patient presents related ocular symptoms and clinical examination shows retrobulbar disease, CT is often the first investigation performed.
2. MRI: Once the CT scan reveals a mass image in the optic nerve area, MRI can be further performed to clarify the nature of the lesions, involving the origin and scope.

10.3.3 *Imaging Findings*

1. CT findings: On CT, ONSM appears as a mass along the optic nerve in isodensity just as soft tissue (Fig. 10.4a, b), and about 20% of mass shows linear or sheetlike calcification. Coronal CT shows an annular hyperdensity image surrounding the optic nerve. If the intracanalicular portion of the optic nerve is involved, the optic canal widening and bony hyperostosis can be seen.
2. MRI findings: The tumor appears iso- to hypointense on T1-weighted images (Figs. 10.4c and 10.5a), and iso- to hypointense on T2-weighted images (Figs. 10.4d and 10.5b). The lesion is enhanced with gadolinium whereas the optic nerve is not, resulting in the typical "double-track sign" (Fig. 10.5c) and "cuff sign" (Figs. 10.4f and 10.5d). Enhanced MRI can also show if the lesion involves the intracranial tissue backward through the optic canal.

10.3.4 *Comments*

CT findings of a mass with calcification along the optic nerve area generally confirm the diagnosis of the ONSM, but for lesions with no calcification, it is hard to differentiate from the optic nerve glioma.

MRI can not only show the range of the lesion, but also help make primary diagnosis based on the characteristic "double-track sign" and "cuff sign" (Shapey et al. 2013).

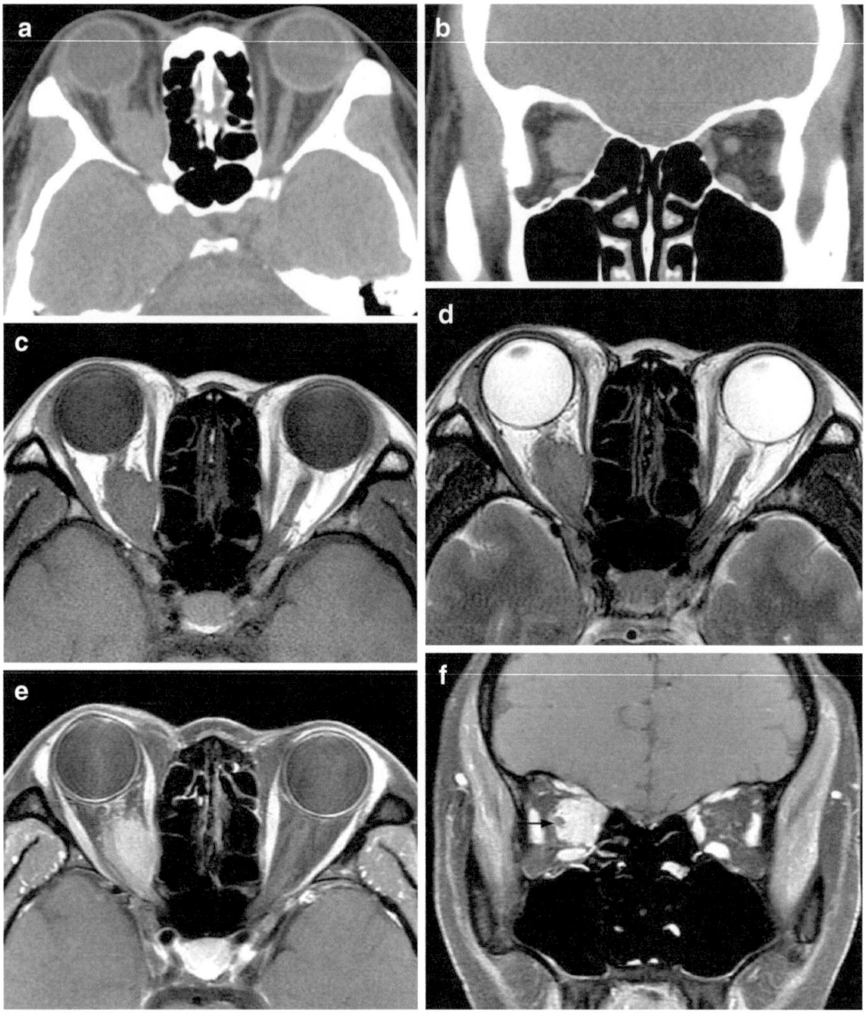

Fig. 10.4 Right optic nerve sheath meningioma. (**a**) Cross-sectional CT soft-tissue window shows that the tumor, displacing the optic nerve laterally, is usually isoattenuating to the soft tissue. (**b**) Coronal CT soft-tissue window shows that the optic nerve is encased by the tumor and the boundary is not clear. (**c**) Cross-sectional T1-weighted MRI shows that the tumor is isointense and has a smooth contour. (**d**) Cross-sectional T2-weighted MRI shows that the mass is isointense and homogeneous. (**e**) Cross-sectional, fat-suppressed, postcontrast MRI image reveals that the tumor, significantly enhanced, surrounds the optic nerve. (**f**) Coronal, fat-suppressed, postcontrast MRI image shows the enhancing tumor around the non-enhancing optic nerve (*arrow*), appearing as the "cuff sign"

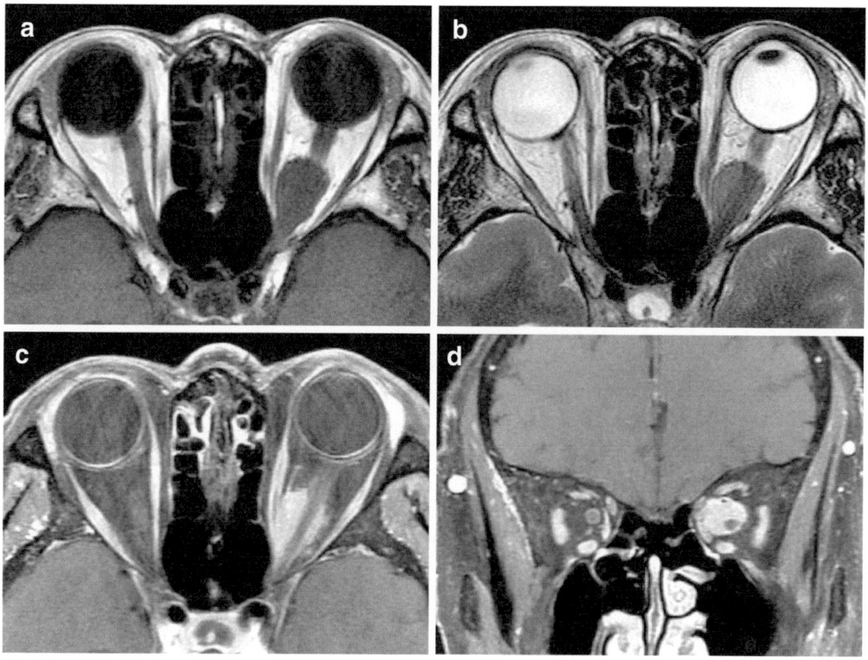

Fig. 10.5 Left optic nerve sheath meningioma. (**a**) Cross-sectional T1-weighted non-enhanced MRI shows that the isointense fusiform tumor grows backward along the optic nerve in the left orbit. (**b**) Cross-sectional T2-weighted MRI shows the mass is isointense and homogeneous; (**c**) Cross-sectional, fat-suppressed, postcontrast MRI image shows the enhancing tumor surrounding the non-enhancing optic nerve, resulting in the "double-track sign." (**d**) Coronal, fat-suppressed, postcontrast MRI image reveals the enhancing tumor around the non-enhancing optic nerve (*arrow*), appearing as the "cuff sign"

10.4 Chiasm Lesions

10.4.1 Pathological Characteristics

Chiasm lesions can be classified as the primary lesion, the secondary, and the congenital chiasm disorder.

10.4.2 The Choice of Imaging Modality

1. MRI is optimal for showing chiasm lesions and should be the first-choice exam when the diagnosis is suspected.
2. CT can show the density feature of the lesion as a supplement, which provides more information for making a diagnosis.

10.4.3 Imaging Findings

1. Imaging characteristics of chiasm lesions include the size, morphology, density, and signal anomaly of the chiasm; mass with abnormal density or signal in the chiasm or its surrounding areas; suprasellar cistern abnormalities such as deformation or occlusion; lower front of the third ventricle deformed, etc.
2. The most common primary tumor of the optic chiasm is gliomas, appearing as a round or an oval mass, occasionally in an irregular shape. The simultaneous presence of enlarged optic nerve and/or optic tract is of significance to the diagnosis of chiasmal gliomas (Fig. 10.6). The tumor can be solid, cystic, or both. The solid components may be contrast enhanced while the cystic may not. Other chiasm tumors such as meningioma, lymphoma, and metastatic tumors are rare.
3. Inflammation of the optic chiasm, or chiasmal optic neuritis, is a demyelinating disorder, most commonly seen in the multiple sclerosis and may coexist with the optic neuritis. The chiasm can be widened or in a normal shape on the imaging, with hyperintensity on T2WI (Fig. 10.7), and varying degrees of contrast enhancement.
4. The secondary chiasm disorder often results from the sellar tumors or mass lesions, among which pituitary tumor is most common. It can cause varying degrees of compression to the optic chiasm (Fig. 10.8). Other lesions include craniopharyngioma, meningioma, Rathke cyst, ICA cavernous aneurysms, empty sella, etc.
5. The congenital chiasm disorder is more associated with other congenital malformations such as septo-optic dysplasia and anophthalmia. Both CT and MRI can reveal the absent or thinning optic chiasm, as well as other malformations.

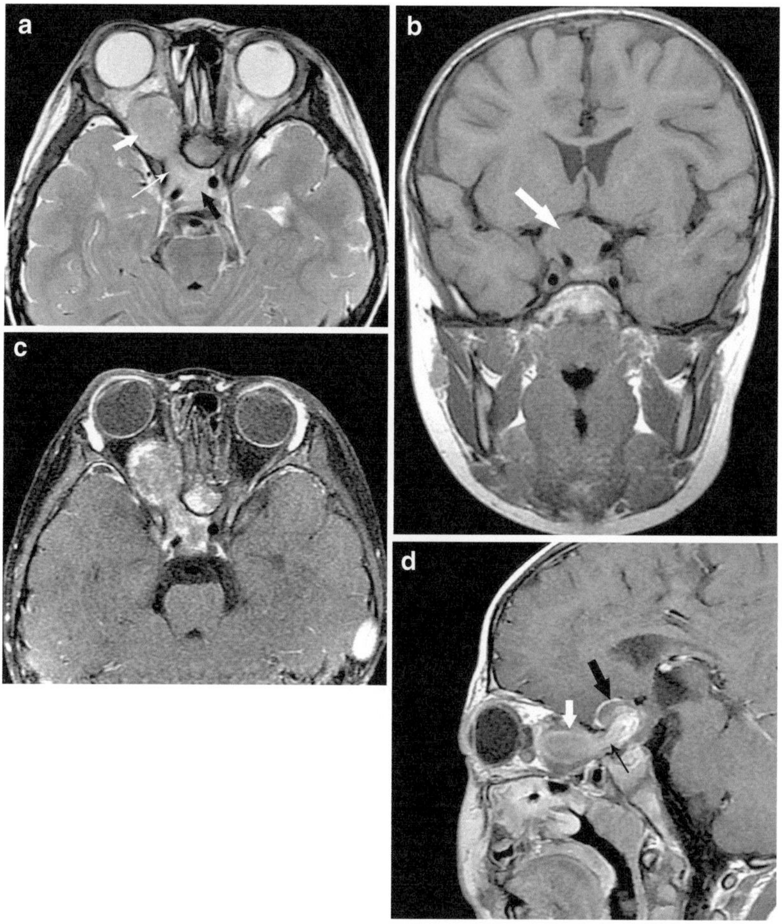

Fig. 10.6 Chiasmal glioma. (**a**) Cross-sectional T2-weighted MRI shows an oval hyperintense mass in the right orbit (*short white arrow*), involving the chiasm backward through the widening optic canal (*long white arrow*), and a heterogeneous hyperintense mass in the chiasmal region (*black arrow*). (**b**) Coronal T1-weighted MRI shows an irregular homogeneous isointense chiasmal mass (*white arrow*). (**c**) Axial, fat-suppressed, postcontrast MRI image shows a lesion with heterogeneous enhancement. (**d**) Oblique sagittal postcontrast MRI image shows an orbital mass (*white arrow*), an optic canal mass (*thin black arrow*), and a chiasmal mass (*thick black arrow*) in the dumbbell shape with heterogeneous enhancement

10.4.4 Comments

MRI is optimal for detecting chiasm lesions. It clearly shows the primary, secondary, and congenital abnormalities and provides evidence for clinical diagnosis of visual impairment. For some lesions, a CT scan may give additional information such as identifying the adjacent bone changes or calcifications within the lesion, and therefore facilitate an accurate diagnosis of the disease.

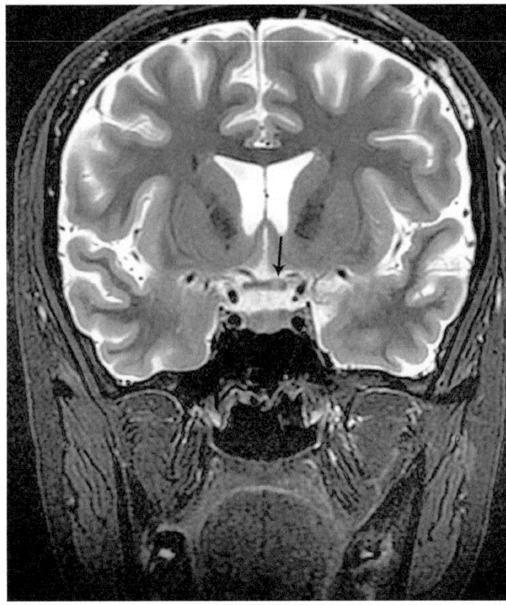

Fig. 10.7 Inflammation of the optic chiasm. Coronal, short time inversion recovery (STIR) MRI image demonstrates that the left side of the chiasm is enlarged and appears hyperintense (*black arrow*)

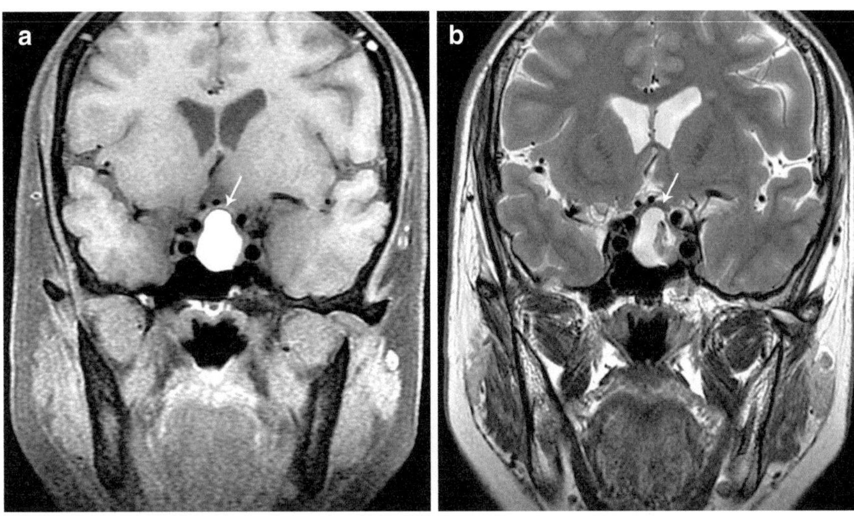

Fig. 10.8 Pituitary *apoplexy* with compression of the optic chiasm. (**a**) Coronal, T1-weighted fat-suppressed MRI image shows an oval-shaped hyperintense mass in the pituitary fossa, compressing and deforming the chiasm upward (*white arrow*). (**b**) Coronal T2-weighted MRI shows dishomogeneous signal intensity within the mass and the elevated chiasm (*white arrow*)

10.5 The Optic Tract Lesions and the Posterior Visual Pathway Lesions

10.5.1 Pathological Characteristics

Primary lesion of the optic tract is rare; it is usually more involved with the adjacent structure abnormalities, including tumors (in the sellar region, third ventricle), aneurysms (in the posterior communicating artery, posterior cerebral artery), vessel occlusion, and meningitis.

The posterior visual pathway lesions mainly include the vascular lesions, vascular malformations, glioma, metastatic tumors, and inflammatory and demyelinating diseases.

10.5.2 The Choice of Imaging Modality

1. MRI, first choice for detecting the optic tract lesions and the posterior visual pathway lesions, can clearly show the site of the lesion and its signal features.
2. A CT exam is quick and convenient. It can show the presence and location of a lesion when MRI is not available.

10.5.3 Imaging Findings

1. Vascular diseases: Infarct is the most common disorder in the occipital lobe, appearing as minimal patchy hypoattenuation on CT (Fig. 10.9a), which can be quite obscure in the acute stage. MRI can detect early ischemic lesions, which shows an area of hyperintensity in the diffuse-weighted imaging (Fig. 10.9b). The infarct lesion turns hypointense on the T1-weighted imaging and hyperintense on the T2-weighted imaging over time (Fig. 10.9c, d), and gyriform enhancement can be seen. In the chronic stage, the lesion becomes softening and is isointense to CSF. Hemorrhage is patchy hyperattenuation on CT (Fig. 10.10). MRI can show the typical three phases of intracranial hemorrhage (ICH): ICH in the acute stage appears as low signal intensity on T2; high signal intensity on T1 and T2 in the subacute stage; low signal intensity on T1; and high signal intensity on T2.
2. Vascular malformations mainly include arteriovenous malformation (AVM) and cavernous hemangioma. MRI can show the tortuous flow voids in AVM. Cavernous hemangioma originated from the visual pathway is quite rare and mostly visual damage is caused by repeated hemorrhage, appearing as hypointense ring around the lesion on MRI (Fig. 10.11).

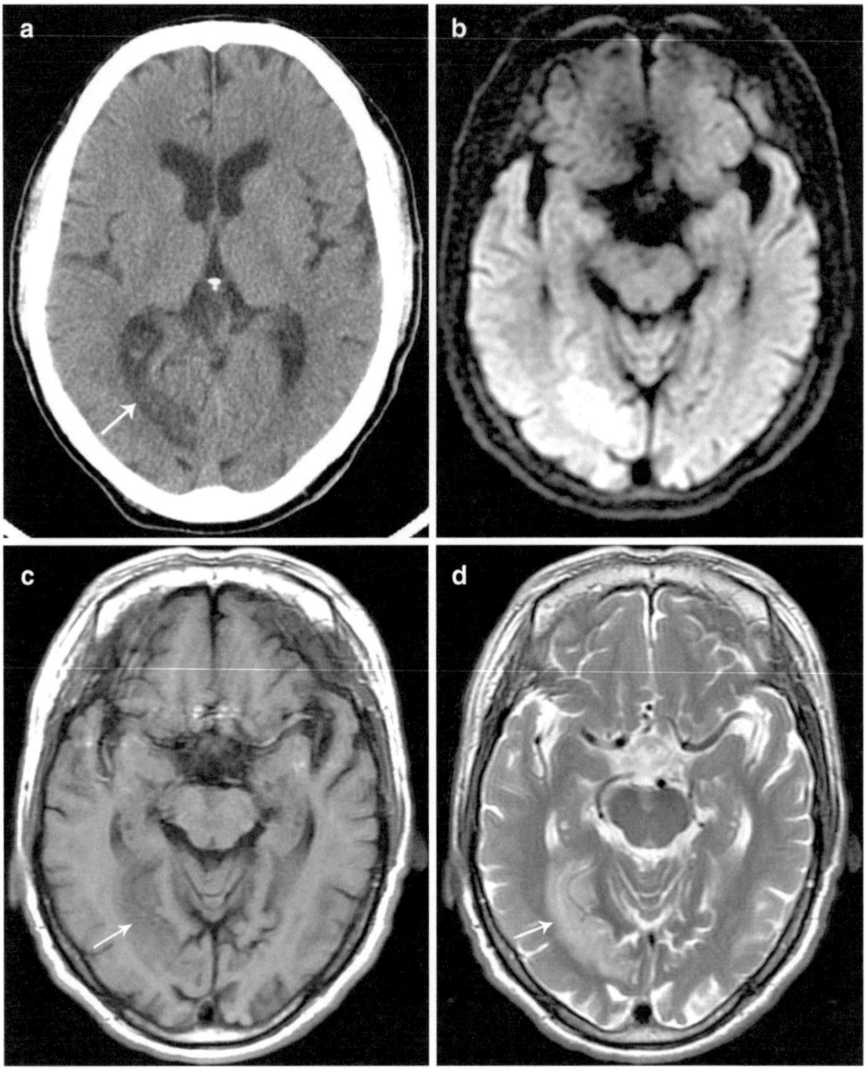

Fig. 10.9 Infarct in the right occipital lobe. (**a**) Cross-sectional CT shows a poorly defined minimal patchy hypoattenuation in the right occipital region (*white arrow*). (**b**) Cross-sectional diffuse-weighted imaging shows right occipital patchy hyperintensity. (**c**) Cross-sectional non-enhanced T1-weighted MRI shows slight hypointensity in the right occipital lobe (*white arrow*). (**d**) Cross-sectional T2-weighted MRI shows a slightly hyperintense patchy lesion in the right occipital area (*white arrow*)

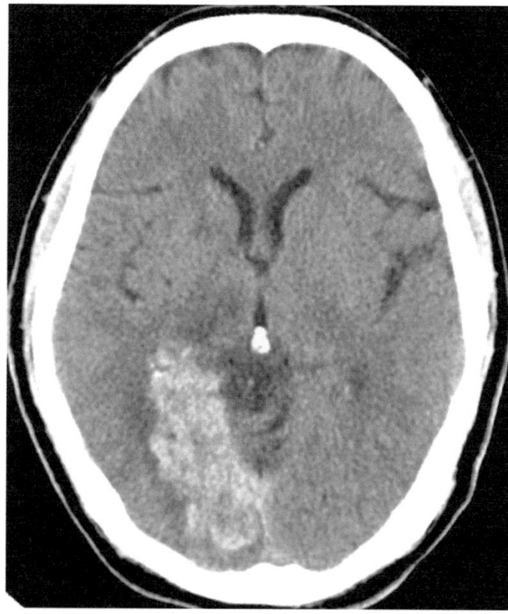

Fig. 10.10 Hemorrhage in the right occipital lobe. Cross-sectional non-enhanced CT shows a well-defined patchy hyperattenuation in the right occipital region

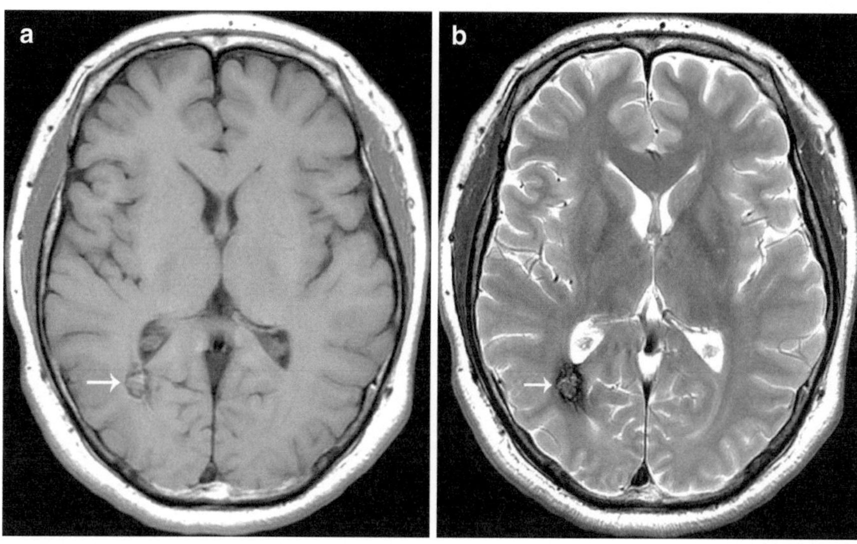

Fig. 10.11 Right occipital cavernous hemangioma. (**a**) Cross-sectional noncontrast T1-weighted MRI shows a quasi-circular right occipital lesion, with slightly higher signal in the center and marginal circular lower signal (*white arrow*). (**b**) Cross-sectional T2-weighted MRI shows a right occipital lesion with a peripheral hypointense rim (*white arrow*)

3. Intracranial aneurysms: Most aneurysms causing visual impairment are located in the distal segment of internal carotid artery, posterior cerebral artery, and posterior communicating artery. They appear as round or quasi-circular minimal hyperattenuation on CT and signal flow void within the aneurysm can be seen on MRI.

10.5.4 Comments

MRI has the advantage of detecting the optic tract lesions and the posterior visual pathway lesions, which can clearly define the location, morphology, and signal features of the lesion and provide a wealth of information for clinical diagnosis. In a few emergency cases such as ICH, CT scan is quick and convenient for initial diagnosis, serving as an effective complement to MRI.

10.6 Ocular Motor Neuropathy

10.6.1 Pathological Characteristics

Ocular motor neuropathy includes the congenital disorders and secondary disorders. The congenital ocular motor neuropathy mainly refers to the abnormality of ocular motor nerve, namely the oculomotor (CN III), trochlear (CN IV), and abducens (CN VI) nerve, and manifest as neurological undeveloped, maldeveloped, or abnormal innervation. The secondary ocular motor neuropathy includes tumor of the nerve itself (e.g., schwannoma), the adjacent aneurysm, compression of the tumor, inflammation of adjacent structures (e.g., Tolosa-Hunt syndrome), traumatic involvement, etc. (Jain et al. 2008).

10.6.2 The Choice of Imaging Modality

1. MRI: MRI is the preferred imaging technique because of its sensitivity in detecting small ocular motor nerve structures.
2. CT: Except detecting traumatic fracture, CT has very limited value to other ocular motor neuropathy.

10.6.3 Imaging Findings

On MRI, undeveloped ocular motor nerve appears as nerve absent (Fig. 10.12), and maldeveloped ocular motor nerve looks slender or absent. What's more, MRI can evaluate the lesions around the ocular motor nerve, such as aneurysms, tumor, and widened cavernous sinus (Fig. 10.13).

10.6.4 Comments

MRI can reveal the abnormal morphology of the ocular motor nerves. For lesions with normal morphology, part of them are enhanced on MRI after administration of contrast gadodiamide. Still some lesions are non-enhanced which cannot be identified through MRI scan.

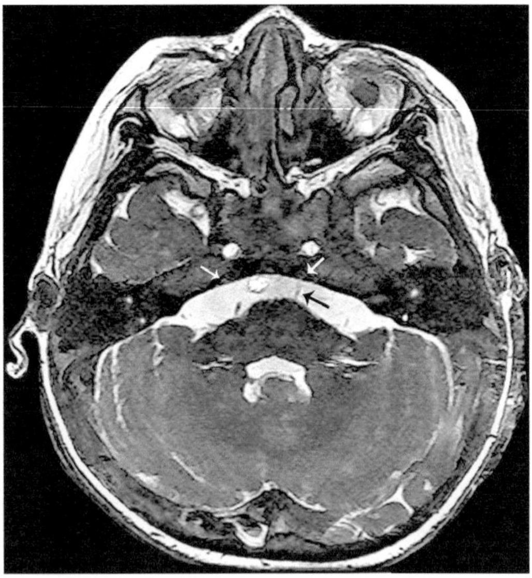

Fig. 10.12 Right abducens nerve hypoplasia. Cross-sectional FIESTA (fast imaging employing steady-state acquisition) MRI shows that the right abducens nerve is absent. The *black arrow* points to the left normal abducens nerve and the *white arrow* points to the bilateral Dorello canals through which the abducens nerves go

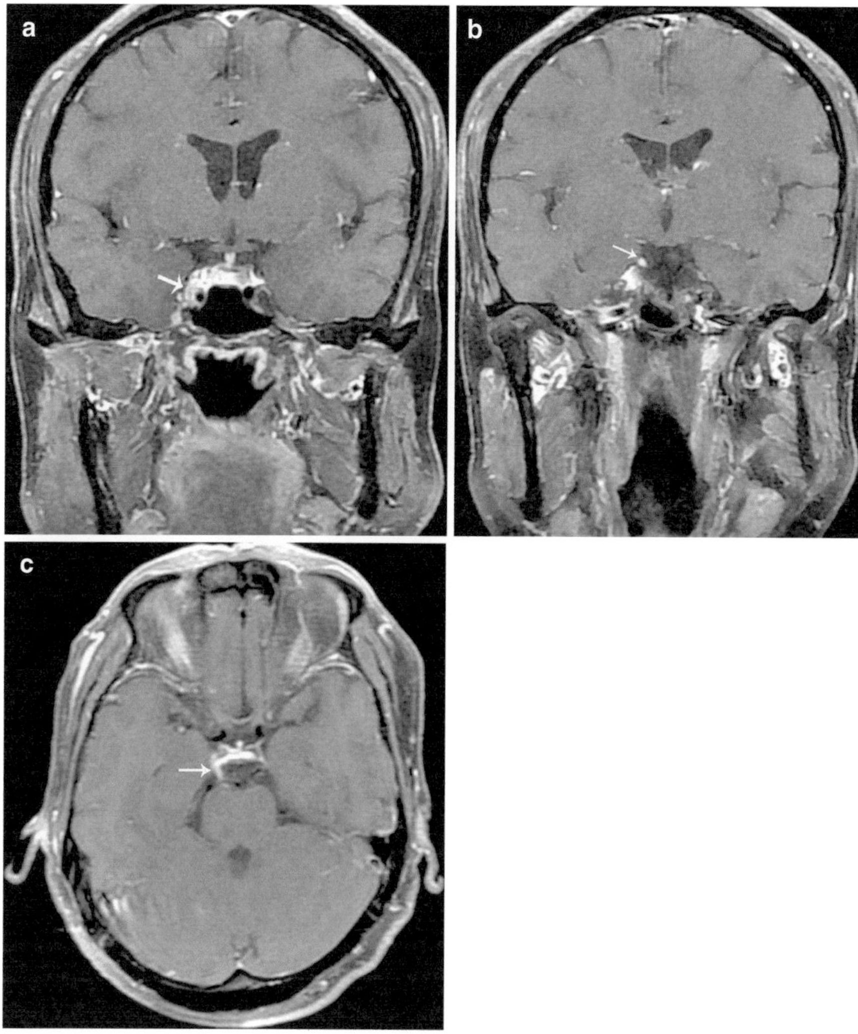

Fig. 10.13 Right cavernous sinus inflammation, involving the right oculomotor nerve. (**a**) Coronal, fat-suppressed, postcontrast MRI image shows the right cavernous sinus is widened and obviously enhanced (*white arrow*). (**b**) Coronal, fat-suppressed, postcontrast MRI image shows the enlarged and significantly enhanced right oculomotor nerve (*white arrow*). (**c**) Cross-sectional, fat-suppressed, postcontrast MRI image shows the enlarged and significantly enhanced right oculomotor nerve (*white arrow*)

10.7 Ocular Sensory Neuropathy

10.7.1 Pathological Characteristics

Ocular sensory neuropathy includes the neoplastic lesions of the branches of the trigeminal nerves and the facial nerves, such as the orbital schwannoma, neurofibroma, neuroblastoma, blood vessels, brain, and trigeminal nerve syndrome (Sturge-Weber syndrome).

10.7.2 The Choice of Imaging Modality

1. CT: A CT scan, the preferred method of examination, can be used to identify the preliminary findings of the presence of lesions.
2. MRI: An MRI scan can be used to perform further diagnosis or when it is necessary to observe the exact extent of disease.

10.7.3 Imaging Findings

For orbital schwannoma or neurofibroma, please refer to the previous chapters.

Neuroblastoma in the orbital socket is mostly a secondary finding, formed from the celiac primary tumor metastases. Imaging performed shows the destruction of the orbital wall bone, visible radial bone needles, and surrounding irregular soft-tissue mass, inhomogeneously marked in the enhanced MRI (Fig. 10.14).

Sturge-Weber syndrome causes a patient to suffer from facial hemangioma along the distribution of the trigeminal nerve (the ophthalmic branch and the maxillary branch) (Fig. 10.15) (Cakirer et al. 2005).

10.7.4 Comments

A CT scan can show the relationship between small schwannomas located in adjacent structures with relative clarity. However, they can be difficult to distinguish when the tumor is large, since the density of the tumor is similar to the density of adjacent structures, so orbital tumors can be difficult to identify.

An MRI can clearly show the relationship between the tumor and the adjacent structures, so it is an easy way to identify orbital tumors, which is helpful for a preliminary diagnosis.

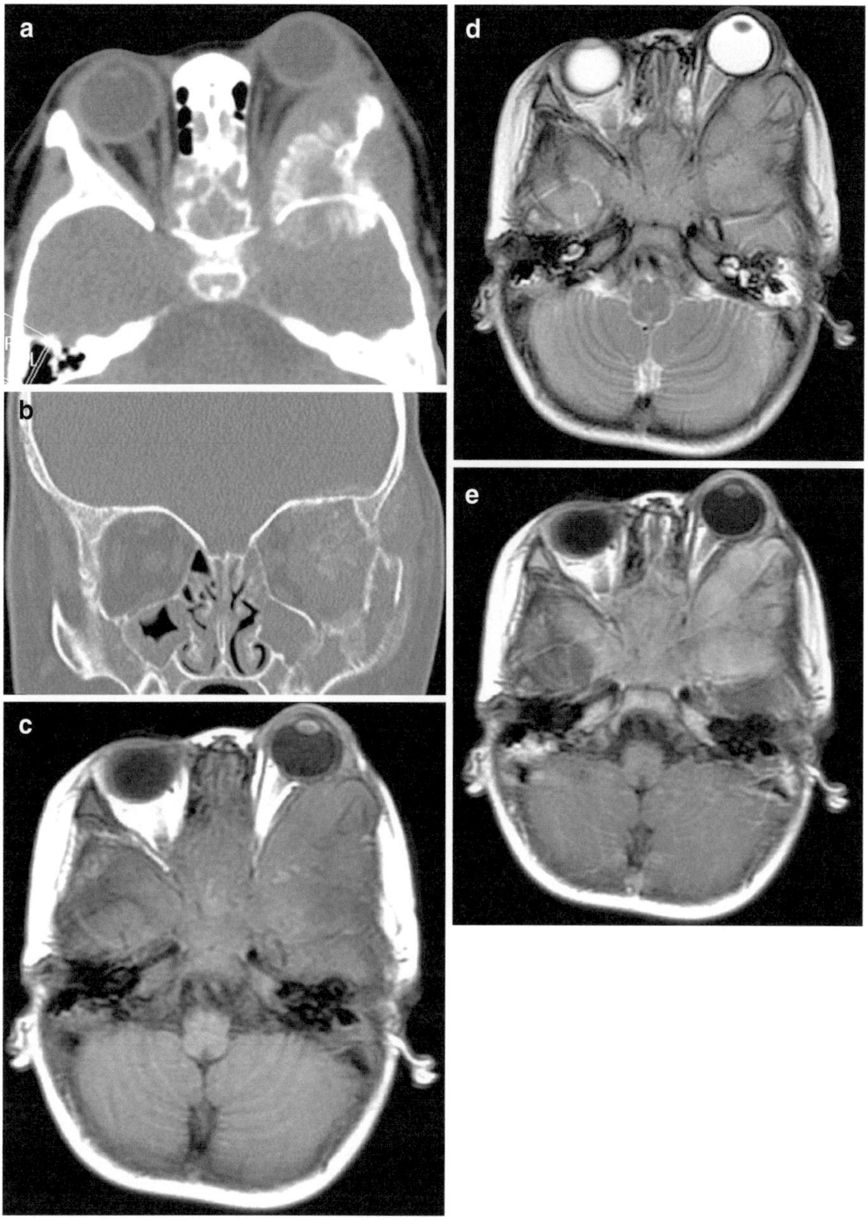

Fig. 10.14 Neuroblastoma with skull base and orbit metastasis. (**a**) Cross-sectional CT soft-tissue window shows a poorly defined soft-tissue mass involving the left lateral orbital wall, with radial high-density shadow inside. (**b**) Coronal CT bone window shows coarse edge of the bone cortex in the lateral and upper wall of the left orbit, with patchy and radial high density shadow in the adjacent soft tissue. (**c**) Cross-sectional T1-weighted MRI shows an ill-defined irregular isointense soft-tissue mass originating from bone of the anterior and middle cranial fossa, involving the left orbit, and compressing the left eyeball, leading to protopsis. (**d**) Cross-sectional T2-weighted MRI shows that the lesion is slightly hyperintense. (**e**) Cross-sectional postcontrast MRI shows that the lesion is significantly enhanced

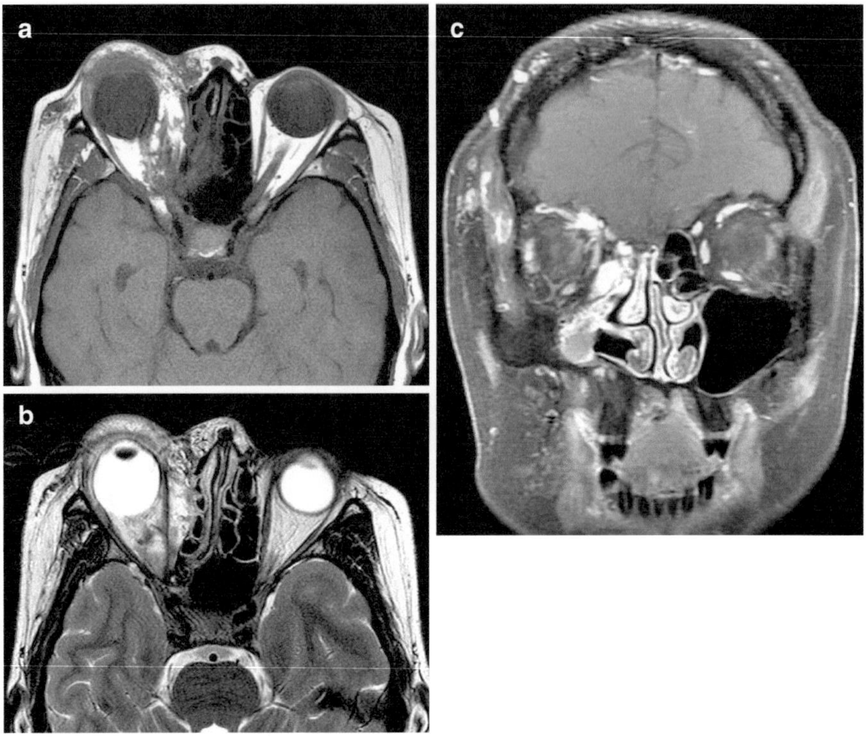

Fig. 10.15 Sturge-Weber syndrome. (**a**) Cross-sectional T1-weighted MRI shows isointense irregular lesion in the right orbit and sporadic isointense angiomatous malformation image in the right eyelid, inner canthus, and temporal fossa. (**b**) Cross-sectional T2-weighted MRI shows a heterogeneous hyperintense lesion with flow voids within. (**c**) Coronal, fat-suppressed, postcontrast MRI image shows intense enhancement of the lesion in the right orbital and frontotemporal soft tissues

References

Cakirer S, Yagmurlu B, Savas MR. Sturge-Weber syndrome: diffusion magnetic resonance imaging and proton magnetic resonance spectroscopy findings. Acta Radiol. 2005;46(4):407–10.

Jain R, Sawhney S, Kou RL, et al. Tolosa-Hunt syndrome: MRI appearances. J Med Imaging Radiat Oncol. 2008;52(5):447–51.

Shams PN, Plant GT. Optic neuritis: a review. Int MS J/MS Forum. 2009;16(3):82–9.

Shapey J, Sabin HI, Danesh-Meyer HV, et al. Diagnosis and management of optic nerve sheath meningiomas. J Clin Neurosci. 2013;20(8):1045–56.

Walrath JD, Engelbert M, Kazim M. Magnetic resonance imaging evidence of optic nerve glioma progression into and beyond the optic chiasm. Ophthal Plast Reconstr Surg. 2008;24(6):473–5.

MIX
Papier aus verantwortungsvollen Quellen
Paper from responsible sources
FSC® C105338

If you have any concerns about our products,
you can contact us on
ProductSafety@springernature.com

In case Publisher is established outside the EU,
the EU authorized representative is:
Springer Nature Customer Service Center GmbH
Europaplatz 3, 69115 Heidelberg, Germany

Printed by Libri Plureos GmbH
in Hamburg, Germany